Osteoporosis, Osteoarthritis and Rheumatoid Arthritis: An Agonizing Skeletal Triad

Edited by

Puneetpal Singh

Department of Human Genetics
Punjabi University
Patiala, Punjab
India

Osteoporosis, Osteoarthritis and Rheumatoid Arthritis: An Agonizing Skeletal Triad

Editor: Puneetpal Singh

ISBN (Online): 978-981-5196-08-5

ISBN (Print): 978-981-5196-09-2

ISBN (Paperback): 978-981-5196-10-8

need for a court order if at any point you breach any terms of this License Agreement. In no event will any delay or failure by Bentham Science Publishers in enforcing your compliance with this License Agreement constitute a waiver of any of its rights.

3. You acknowledge that you have read this License Agreement, and agree to be bound by its terms and conditions. To the extent that any other terms and conditions presented on any website of Bentham Science Publishers conflict with, or are inconsistent with, the terms and conditions set out in this License Agreement, you acknowledge that the terms and conditions set out in this License Agreement shall prevail.

Bentham Science Publishers Pte. Ltd.
80 Robinson Road #02-00
Singapore 068898
Singapore
Email: subscriptions@benthamscience.net

BENTHAM
SCIENCE

CONTENTS

PREFACE

This book is about three formidable skeletal diseases; osteoporosis, osteoarthritis and rheumatoid arthritis, which are severely threatening the public health system and increasing the chronic disease burden. Identification and prevention of this agonizing triad are complex, composite and complicated, as several molecular culprits collaborate and contribute to their development and progression. Fragile, flamed and fractured elements of bone affiliated to these disorders have been examined from several perspectives but contradictions and controversies have further amassed to their complexity. This family of skeletal triad has many uninvited and unsolicited related effects in the form of pain, stress and anxiety that their remedial prescriptions to get rid of them become confusing and perplexing. Commoners perceive these health issues either casually or as artefact of misconceived notions and fall prey to unqualified quacks and half-baked practitioners. It is equivocally accepted that there are many underlying mechanisms and mediators that commonly as well as individually influence the pathology of osteoporosis, osteoarthritis and rheumatoid arthritis. Recent scientific work has identified some frightful perpetrators and their *modus operandi* in the initiation, development and progression, but the troubled bones demand further investigations.

The present eBook, "Osteoporosis, Osteoarthritis and Rheumatoid Arthritis: An Agonizing Skeletal Triad" intends to bring together insightful leads on the latest news, views, and reviews from authors, scientists, and clinicians from different regions of the world on these skeletal abnormalities. This compendium is a sincere effort to have input of internationally acclaimed scholars and thinkers to reveal those cellular and molecular culprits who participate but are absconding from the scene of pain and suffering posed to our elderly population afflicting them by these musculoskeletal problems.

In the first chapter, "Osteoporosis and Chronic Liver Disease", the author Yi-Liang Tsai, sheds light on the close inter-relationship of chronic liver disease with osteoporosis. A substantial percentage of chronic liver disease patients suffer from osteoporosis because of disturbed calcium homeostasis. The liver is an important organ that plays a crucial role in several physiological, metabolic and immune-related processes. Composed of hepatocytes, biliary epithelial cells, stellate cells, kupffer cells and hepatic sinusoidal endothelial cells, the liver controls endocrine growth signaling pathways, blood volume regulation, cholesterol homeostasis, nutrient metabolism, and immune system regulation. The role played by the liver in distressed form causing disturbed calcium homeostasis and dysregulated nutrient balance in relation to bone mass has been elaborated on in this chapter.

The second chapter, "Detection of Knee Osteoarthritis using Artificial Intelligence" enriches our knowledge regarding the identification of knee osteoarthritis with artificial intelligence. Knee osteoarthritis is a degenerating joint disorder that affects joints and causes functional disability and pain if left untreated. Therefore, the identification of knee osteoarthritis at an early stage is crucial for better management and prevention, but early identification is complicated, confusing, and sometimes missed. It is envisioned and analysed by Thongpat and co-authors in this chapter that artificial intelligence involving a Convoluted Neural Network (CNN) can predict the early stage of knee osteoarthritis. Such a wonderful effort can substantiate the already existing identification techniques (Kellgren Lawrence grading) from radiographic images that hold a promising future in the direction of better prognosis, diagnosis and therapeutic modalities of knee osteoarthritis.

The third chapter, "Role of Cytokines and Chemokines in Rheumatoid Arthritis" exhibits the details of inflammation, which is the chief culprit in rheumatoid arthritis. Rheumatoid arthritis is a chronic auto-inflammatory disease having progressive cartilage deterioration, synovial inflammation and periarticular calcium erosion. The causes are multifactorial and complex which have fostered diverse therapeutic modalities for its remission, which is possible but challenging because of heterogeneous symptoms, late referrals, or mimicking with other pathologies. A better understanding of the ways that inflammatory mediators trigger and propagate the deterioration of joints is imperative for developing efficient treatments. In the pursuit of a better understanding of inflammation in rheumatoid arthritis, the role and relevance of cytokines and chemokines must be probed as cellular and molecular determinants. Details of some such pro-inflammatory mediators; tumour-necrosis factor-alpha (TNF-α), interleukin-6 (IL-6), IL-8 along with CC chemokines (CCL2, CCL3, CCL4 and CCL5) and CXC chemokines (CXCL5, CXCL8, CXCL9 and CXCL10) have been reported in this chapter.

The fourth chapter, "Vitamin D and Immune System: Implications in Bone Health" has introduced that the host immune system interacting with vitamin D plays a significant role in maintaining calcium and mineral turnover along with the preservation of bone strength. Vitamin D supplementation helps in absorbing calcium, and bone minerals and has great immunomodulatory potential, which not only serves as a guard against bone resorption but also facilitates healing and repair. The showcasing of the importance of vitamin D through the interaction of the immune system and maintenance of calcium homeostasis within the scenario of osteoimmunology is wonderfully presented.

In the fifth chapter, "Bone Water: Effects of Drugs on Bone Hydration Status", Dr. Khan reviewed an unforeseen but important aspect of bone hydration. Water is a crucial nutrient that constitutes approximately 20 percent of the cortical bone by volume. It influences mechanical properties, agility and quality of bone whereas, bone dehydration can stimulate stress-induced deformity (modulus of elasticity). The ill effects of bone dehydration increase manifold in elderly individual where dehydration of the bone interacts with frailty and cause fragility of the bone leading to susceptibility to fractures. The author has shown that bone dehydration also supplements disease severity and worse outcomes in diseases like diabetes, osteoporosis, and osteogenesis. Drugs also induce hypo-hydration of the bones and the interaction between drugs and bone water *vis-à-vis* skeletal health has been highlighted in this chapter.

The sixth chapter, "Dietary Patterns and Rheumatoid Arthritis" has exhibited the importance and necessity of a balanced diet to resist the formidable pangs of pain and suffering in rheumatoid arthritis. The authors have highlighted different forms of diets and dietary patterns and have explained their pros and cons in the pathology of rheumatoid arthritis. It is proposed that a good balanced diet can regulate the underlying inflammatory and immunomodulatory pathways influencing the disease's severity and its outcome.

Chapter seven," Self-perceived Quality of Life in South Asian and British White Rheumatoid Arthritis Patients in the East Midlands, UK" has investigated the heterogeneity of pain, pain-affiliated disease severity and quality of life in rheumatoid arthritis patients of South Asia and British White residing in East Midlands, UK. The analysis of self-perceived quality of life between these two groups has revealed that reduced mobility and physical activity are associated with higher pain perception in South Asian rheumatoid arthritis patients. Such studies have important implications for setting interventional guidelines for pain-resolving treatment outcomes as an individual's culture, education, financial situation, diet, and family support have a strong impact on pain realization and perception.

I am deeply indebted to Mr. Nitin Kumar and Ms. Srishti Valecha for their extended help in the style editing of the book. I extend my heartfelt gratitude to Ms. Noor ul Ain Khan, Manager Publications, Mr. Obaid Sadiq, Manager, Mrs. Humaira Hashmi, Editorial Manager Publications and especially Mr. Mahmood Alam, Director Publications, Bentham Science Publishers for their kind support, encouragement and help.

Puneetpal Singh
Department of Human Genetics
Punjabi University
Patiala, Punjab
India

DEDICATION

To my loving God, who lovingly gave me two lovable gifts: My Wife and Son

List of Contributors

A. Moorthy Rheumatology, University Hospitals of Leicester NHS Trust, Leicester, United Kingdom

A. Samanta Rheumatology, University Hospitals of Leicester NHS Trust, Leicester, United Kingdom

A.M. Ghelani Human Genetics Lab., School of Sport, Exercise and Health Sciences, Loughborough University, Loughborough, LE11 3TU, United Kingdom

Ali Hojati Department of Community Nutrition, Faculty of Nutrition, Tabriz University of Medical Sciences, Tabriz, East Azerbaijan Province, 5166/15731, Tabriz, Iran

Asha Bhardwaj Translational Immunology, Osteoimmunology & Immunoporosis Lab (TIOIL), Department of Biotechnology, All India Institute of Medical Sciences (AIIMS), New Delhi-110029, India

Chayanin Angthong Faculty of Medicine, King Mongkut's Institute of Technology Ladkrabang (KMITL), Bangkok, Thailand

Hanan Hassan Omar Clinical Pathology Department, Faculty of Medicine, Suez Canal University, Ismailia, Egypt

L. Goh Rheumatology, University Hospitals of Leicester NHS Trust, Leicester, United Kingdom

Leena Sapra Translational Immunology, Osteoimmunology & Immunoporosis Lab (TIOIL), Department of Biotechnology, All India Institute of Medical Sciences (AIIMS), New Delhi-110029, India

Mahdieh Abbasalizad Farhangi Department of Community Nutrition, Faculty of Nutrition, Tabriz University of Medical Sciences, Tabriz, East Azerbaijan Province, 5166/15731, Tabriz, Iran

Mohammad Ahmed Khan Department of Pharmacology, School of Pharmaceutical Education and Research, Jamia Hamdard, New Delhi-110062, India

Napat Pongsakonpruttikul Faculty of Medicine, King Mongkut's Institute of Technology Ladkrabang (KMITL), Bangkok, Thailand

Pongphak Thongpat Faculty of Medicine, King Mongkut's Institute of Technology Ladkrabang (KMITL), Bangkok, Thailand

Puneetpal Singh Department of Human Genetics, Punjabi University, Patiala, Punjab, India

Rupesh K. Srivastava Translational Immunology, Osteoimmunology & Immunoporosis Lab (TIOIL), Department of Biotechnology, All India Institute of Medical Sciences (AIIMS), New Delhi-110029, India

Sarabjit Mastana Human Genetics Lab., School of Sport, Exercise and Health Sciences, Loughborough University, Loughborough, LE11 3TU, United Kingdom

Sneha Das Translational Immunology, Osteoimmunology & Immunoporosis Lab (TIOIL), Department of Biotechnology, All India Institute of Medical Sciences (AIIMS), New Delhi-110029, India

Tamanna Sharma   Translational Immunology, Osteoimmunology & Immunoporosis Lab (TIOIL), Department of Biotechnology, All India Institute of Medical Sciences (AIIMS), New Delhi-110029, India

Tsai Yi-Liang   Department of Nuclear Medicine, Dalin Tzu Chi Hospital, Buddhist Tzu Chi Medical Foundation, Chiayi 622401, Taiwan

CHAPTER 1

Osteoporosis and Chronic Liver Disease

Tsai Yi-Liang[1],*

[1] Department of Nuclear Medicine, Dalin Tzu Chi Hospital, Buddhist Tzu Chi Medical Foundation, Chiayi 622401, Taiwan

Abstract: The liver is composed of hepatocytes, biliary epithelial cells, Kupffer cells, stellate cells, and hepatic sinusoidal endothelial cells. It also plays an important role in the digestive system and immune system at the same time. The different types of hepatitis, including viral liver diseases, autoimmune liver diseases, and metabolic liver diseases, are all closely related to osteoporosis. People with liver disease have a significantly higher risk of developing osteoporosis than people without hepatitis. Fibrosis is part of the wound-healing response that maintains organs after tissue injury, but excessive fibrosis may also contribute to a variety of human diseases. Hepatic stellate cells are the key to liver fibrosis. The apoptotic hepatocytes stimulate fibrosis in hepatic myofibroblasts, and activated hepatic stellate cells are the main source of myofibroblasts in the liver. Activated hepatic stellate cells possess many voltage-operated calcium channels. Changes in the concentration of calcium ions mediate hepatic stellate cell activation and fibrosis regression. The skeleton is one of the main regulatory mechanisms of calcium ions in the body. Therefore, chronic hepatitis leads to a disturbance of calcium homeostasis *in vivo*, which may be one of the factors causing bone loss.

Keywords: Autoimmune liver disease, Bone mineral density, Fibrosis, Metabolic liver disease, Osteoporosis, Viral liver disease.

INTRODUCTION

There are three main causes of osteoporosis caused by chronic kidney disease: abnormal calcium and phosphorus metabolism, vitamin D deficiency, and secondary hyperparathyroidism. Parathyroid hormone (PTH) can activate osteoclasts to break down bone, release calcium ions and increase blood calcium concentration. When PTH acts on the kidney, it helps the kidney to produce vitamin D and increase calcium reabsorption [1, 2]. Low vitamin D levels stimulate PTH production, but high vitamin D levels do not always lead to low

---
* **Corresponding author Tsai Yi-Liang:** Department of Nuclear Medicine, Dalin Tzu Chi Hospital, Buddhist Tzu Chi Medical Foundation, Chiayi 622401, Taiwan; Tel: +886-4-7238595 #4971; E-mail: 5l4vupm6@gmail.com

Puneetpal Singh (Ed.)

PTH levels. Serum PTH levels will be low and stable when vitamin D is above 30 ng/mL [3 - 5].

Both chronic kidney disease and chronic hepatitis are known to increase the risk of osteoporosis. The common causes are disturbed calcium metabolism and vitamin D deficiency.

The liver is an important organ that maintains the normal life activities of the body and is a key hub for many physiological processes. It is composed of hepatocytes, biliary epithelial cells, stellate cells, Kupffer cells, and hepatic sinusoidal endothelial cells. Its functions include controlling endocrine growth signaling pathways, blood volume regulation, lipid and cholesterol homeostasis, breakdown of exogenous compounds, and nutrient metabolism (carbohydrates, lipids and proteins) [6].

In addition, the liver plays an important role in the immune system. Overexpressed inflammation leads to tissue damage and remodeling, and chronic inflammation when immunity is compromised [7]. In chronic liver disease, viral, toxic, metabolic, or autoimmune triggers lead to hepatocyte death, followed by inflammation and compensatory proliferation, associated with the development of fibrosis, cirrhosis, and even hepatocellular carcinoma [8].

OSTEOPOROSIS & LIVER DISEASES

Vitamin D not only plays an important role in regulating bone, calcium, and phosphate metabolism [9], but also plays a key role in liver diseases. Vitamin D deficiency is often observed in chronic liver diseases, including hepatitis B virus [10, 11], hepatitis C virus [12, 13], and non-alcoholic fatty liver disease [14, 15]. Osteoporosis is a common complication in patients with chronic liver disease, with a prevalence ranging from approximately 4% to 21% [16]. It is currently known that liver diseases predisposing to osteoporosis include viral liver diseases (hepatitis B and hepatitis C), autoimmune liver diseases (ALD) (autoimmune hepatitis (AH), primary biliary cirrhosis (PBC), and sclerosing cholangitis) and metabolic liver diseases (alcoholic hepatitis and non-alcoholic fatty liver disease).

Viral Liver Disease

Both hepatitis B virus (HBV) and hepatitis C virus (HCV) are hepatotropic viruses. HBV is a partly double-stranded DNA virus [17]; HCV is a single-stranded RNA virus [18]. The main route of infection is the virus-infected blood and body fluids entering human body, through the skin or mucous membranes, especially the blood.

Hepatitis B Virus

The cross-sectional study of Chen *et al.* assessed the association between the patients with HBV infection and bone mineral density (BMD) using a multiple linear regression model. The covariates are age, gender, body mass index, proteinuria, serum total cholesterol, uric acid, creatinine, glutamic-oxaloacetic transaminase, albumin, C-reactive protein, thyrotropin, history of smoking and drinking. The results of the fully adjusted model have shown that HBV infection is significantly negatively correlated with BMD (β= -0.17, $p<0.05$) [19].

Another 12-year longitudinal study has assessed the association between HBV infection and osteoporosis risk. Of 180,730 patients admitted, 36,146 and 144,584 patients were divided into an HBV-infected group and a control group, respectively. The factors adjusted in the model included age, gender, frequency of hospital visits, hypertension, diabetes, hyperlipidemia, heart failure, liver cirrhosis, chronic kidney disease, thyroid disease, steroid drugs, warfarin, proton pump inhibitor, aspirin and estrogen replacement therapy. Compared with the control group, the HBV-infected group had a 1.13-fold higher risk of developing osteoporosis [20].

In the terms of vitamin D, low serum $25(OH)D_3$ levels are associated with high levels of HBV replication in patients with chronic hepatitis B [21]. HBV can utilize multiple mechanisms to increase intracellular Ca^{2+} concentration, creating a cellular environment to facilitate its infection [22].

A prospective study by Mohamed *et al.* has reported a change in serum $25(OH)D_3$ levels in chronic hepatitis B patients before and during antiviral therapy. A total of 50 treatment-naive chronic HBV patients and 30 healthy subjects were enrolled in the study. The cases received treatment in the form of Lamivudine 100 mg tablet, once daily. Serum $25(OH)D_3$ levels were assessed twice, once before initiation of antiviral treatment and again at least 6 months later. The studied cases showed significantly low mean serum vitamin D levels when assessed before treatment (21.6 ± 5.8 ng/ml) as compared to the levels after 6 months of treatment (31.1 ± 7.3 ng/ml) which was comparable to that of the control group (33.4 ± 5 ng/ml) [23].

Hepatitis C Virus

69 chronic HCV-infected participants were enrolled in a prospective cohort study. The results showed that the mean BMD, Z-score, and T-score of the lumbar spine in patients with chronic hepatitis C were significantly lower than the control group without chronic hepatitis C ($p<0.001$). The results also showed that bone alkaline phosphatase and the C-terminal cross-linked telopeptide of type I

collagen were significantly elevated in chronic hepatitis C patients with reduced BMD [24]. The findings are similar to those of Lai *et al.* Procollagen type I amino-terminal pro-peptide, one of the bone turnover biomarkers [25, 26], is useful in identifying chronic HCV patients at increased risk of bone loss [27].

Vitamin D not only plays an important role in calcium metabolism [25, 28], but also acts as an immune modulator. It can reduce inflammation while enhancing protective immune responses [29]. Gutierrez *et al.* have shown that bone loss in HCV patients is related to the high prevalence of 25-hydroxyvitamin D deficiency [29]. Moreover, low vitamin D level has been associated with high hepatic necro-inflammatory activity and progression of liver fibrosis, and it can affect the response to antiviral therapy in HCV patients [30].

Autoimmune Liver Diseases

Autoimmune liver diseases are caused by immune-mediated damage to tissues. Autoimmune liver disease and rheumatic disease coexist in approximately 30% of cases and may share a common pathogenic mechanism [31]. The common autoimmune liver diseases, with a high risk of osteoporosis, include primary biliary cholangitis (PBC) and autoimmune hepatitis (AIH) targeting hepatocytes.

Primary Biliary Cholangitis

PBC is an autoimmune cholestatic liver disease clinically characterized by bile duct destruction, sometimes with granulomas. Osteoporosis is a common complication of PBC [32]. It mainly affects middle-aged women and is characterized by chronic progressive destruction of small intrahepatic bile ducts, with portal inflammation and eventual fibrosis [33]. Osteoporosis is more common in women with PBC than in the general population. Age and disease severity are major risk factors for osteoporosis in PBC, but are not associated with menopausal status [34]. At present, the pathogenesis of PBC is not well known, but it is mainly due to low bone formation [35]. Therefore, the American Association for the Study of Liver Disease has recommended that the treatment of PBC can use vitamin D, calcium supplementation, and alendronate to increase bone mass effectively and to prevent bone loss [36].

The best form of vitamin D for PBC is calcitriol because it is the active form of the vitamin D3 metabolite. Its receptors are present in sinusoidal endothelial cells, Kupffer cells, and stellate cells of normal liver, as well as cholangiocyte lineages [37]. The study by Wang *et al.* measured the serum vitamin D levels in 185 PBC patients in which patients with late-stage PBC had lower mean vitamin D levels (9.15 ± 5.33 ng/ml) than patients with early-stage PBC (13.68 ± 6.33 ng/ml) ($p < 0.001$). Vitamin D levels tended to rise in patients taking calcitriol, as compared to those who were not taking calcitriol (p = 0.027). In addition, vitamin D-deficient PBC patients have higher bilirubin and lower albumin [38]. Also of interest, seasonal changes in PBC may be partly related to vitamin D. From 1987 to 2003 in the North East of England, a clear peak in the local diagnosis of PBC was observed in June, but the mechanism has not yet been understood [39].

Autoimmune Hepatitis

AIH shows prominent portal and lobular lymphoplasmacytic inflammation [40]. AIH is a rare autoimmune disease, about 5% of all chronic liver diseases. It is characterized by female predominance, hypergammaglobulinemia, extrahepatic syndrome and favorable response to immunosuppressive therapy [41].

Osteoporosis is a common complication of AIH. A study has shown that almost 20% of AIH patients with age greater than 50 years have osteoporosis. Aging, duration of corticosteroid use, low body mass index, and liver fibrosis are independent risk factors for bone loss [42].

The 25(OH)D deficiency plays an important role in predicting AIH severity *via* inflammatory cytokine production. A study investigates 66 AIH patients (7 males, 59 females), the results of which indicate that serum total 25(OH)D levels are significantly lower in patients with acute-onset AIH than in patients with chronic-onset AIH. Serum total 25(OH)D levels are significantly reduced in patients with severe AIH [43]. Another study also shows that unresponsiveness to treatment is more common in patients with severe vitamin D deficiency (59%) than in patients without deficiency (41%) (p = 0.04). Moreover, severe vitamin D deficiency is also independently associated with a higher risk of developing cirrhosis (hazard ratio = 3.40, p = 0.01), and liver-related mortality or requirement for liver transplantation (hazard ratio = 5.26, p = 0.008) [44].

Metabolic Liver Diseases

Metabolic liver diseases can be divided into alcoholic liver disease (ALD) and non-alcoholic fatty liver disease (NAFLD), the latter is also called metabolic-associated fatty liver disease (MAFLD).

Alcoholic Liver Disease

The liver is the main organ responsible for metabolizing ethanol [45]. The alcohol metabolism would generate reactive oxygen species. These active radicals are usually produced by the mitochondria, endoplasmic reticulum or Kupffer cells. These rapidly form a variety of active metabolites which can further contribute to oxidative stress in hepatocytes [46].

Alcohol intake is an important factor in the development of osteoporosis, but moderate drinking can reduce fracture rates and increase BMD. The study has shown that BMD is higher in men and postmenopausal women, who drink alcohol as compared to those who refrain from it. Drinking alcohol in moderate amount appears to be beneficial to bone health [47]. It has a good effect on high-density lipoprotein cholesterol levels and has an inhibitory effect on platelet aggregation [48]. In addition, suitable alcohol consumption may help to maintain bone density in postmenopausal women by increasing endogenous estrogens or promoting the secretion of calcitonin [49].

Acute alcoholism causes transient hypoparathyroidism, leading to hypocalcemia and hypercalciuria. However, long-term moderate alcohol consumption increases serum PTH levels. Chronic alcoholics are characterized by low serum vitamin D metabolite levels, leading to calcium malabsorption, hypocalcemia, and hypocalciuria [50]. This finding is consistent with the idea that moderate alcohol consumption increases BMD but excessive drinking decreases BMD.

However, there has been no consensus so far on how much amount of alcohol is to be considered moderate. The study by de Lorimier has suggested that it should not exceed 2 to 4 drinks per day for men, and 1 to 2 drinks per day for women [48]. The male subjects in a study population of Tucker *et al.* are predominantly beer drinkers. The results show that alcohol intake in men greater than 2 glasses per day is associated with significantly lower BMD [51]. Feskanich *et al.* recommend that the weekly alcohol intake should be less than 75 grams [49].

Although drinking alcohol has inconsistent effects on bones, it is one of the causes of osteoporosis [52]. Chronic alcoholic patients are frequently deficient in one or more vitamins, including folate, vitamin B6, thiamine, vitamin A and vitamin D [53, 54]. 90% of patients with alcoholic cirrhosis have vitamin D deficiency (80nmol/L) [54]. The pathogenesis of loss of BMD in ALD is multifactorial, including the toxic effects of alcohol on bone and endocrine, nutritional disturbances secondary to alcoholism and deficiencies in osteocalcin, vitamin D and insulin growth factor-1. These factors may be the result of imbalances in bone formation and resorption [55].

Metabolic Associated Fatty Liver Disease

Metabolic-associated fatty liver disease (MAFLD) is considered a more appropriate overall term than non-alcoholic fatty liver disease (NAFLD) as the latter does not reflect the heterogeneity of fatty liver disease pathogenesis, and the inaccuracy of terminology and definitions necessitates a re-evaluation of nomenclature to inform clinical trial design and drug development [56].

MAFLD is a clinicopathological syndrome closely associated with obesity, inflammation and insulin resistance, characterized by excessive lipid deposition in hepatocytes [56, 57].

The cross-sectional analysis of 231 asymptomatic subjects, of which, 129 subjects have MAFLD, reveals that BMD of the lumbar spine, femur neck and total hip is significantly lower in MAFLD patients with significant fibrosis, compared with MAFLD patients without significant fibrosis. The multivariate linear regression model, after adjustment for age, gender, body mass index, alanine amino-transferase, high-density lipoprotein cholesterol, fasting plasma glucose, and liver steatosis, disclosed that liver fibrosis is independently correlated with low BMD at the femur neck ($\beta = -0.18$, $p = 0.039$) and total hip ($\beta = -0.21$, $p = 0.005$). Furthermore, using multivariable logistic regression, the results indicate that the presence of liver fibrosis is significantly associated with an increased risk for overall low bone mass and osteoporosis in MAFLD subjects (odds ratio = 4.10) [58]. Another study conducted on children has shown similar results [59].

To see the effect of vitamin D supplementation, in a small double-blind placebo-controlled study in MAFLD subjects, the participants are randomly assigned to the group with vitamin D supplementation (50,000 IU every 14 days for 4 months) and the control group (no vitamin D supplementation). After 4 months, the results have shown that the improved vitamin D status leads to amelioration in serum high-sensitive C-reactive protein and malondialdehyde (markers of lipid peroxidation) in patients with MAFLD [60]. In a large study with 12,878 subjects, 4,027 have been diagnosed with MAFLD, accounting for 31.27% of the total population; 5,895 patients have vitamin D deficiency, accounting for 45.78% of the total population. Multivariate analysis has shown that vitamin D insufficiency is an independent risk factor for MAFLD after adjustment with other confounders (odds ratio = 1.130) [61]. In another large cross-sectional study, a total of 83,625 subjects were enrolled. Multivariate linear regression analysis model after adjusting for the risk factors also finds a negative correlation between the serum vitamin D levels and MAFLD (odds ratio = 0.92, $p = 0.001$) [62].

Several factors may increase the risk of osteoporosis in MAFLD. These include the release of cytokines from the inflamed liver which may influence the bone microenvironment, vitamin D deficiency, and limited physical activity. Circulating markers of bone metabolism, including osteopontin, osteoprotegerin, osteocalcin and fetuin-A, have been found to be altered in patients with MAFLD [63].

Liver Fibrosis and Bone

Liver fibrosis is the result of the wound-healing response to repeated injury [64]. Fibrosis occurs as part of the wound-healing response to maintain organ integrity after tissue damage, but excessive fibrosis can also contribute to a variety of human diseases, such as liver cirrhosis [65, 66].

Hepatic stellate cells are the critical target in liver fibrosis [67]. Quiescent hepatic stellate cells are located in the space of Disse [65]. Several cellular events in inflamed hepatic tissue microenvironment as well as extrahepatic factors are known to directly induce hepatic stellate cell activation in etiology-specific or independent manner, for example, epithelial cell injury, altered extracellular matrix, immune regulation, metabolic dysregulation, enteric dysbiosis and chronic infection of hepatitis virus [68]. The apoptotic hepatocytes will stimulate fibrosis in hepatic myofibroblasts [69], whereas activated hepatic stellate cells are the main source of myofibroblasts in the liver [70].

In response to liver injury, hepatic stellate cells undergo marked morphological and functional changes, from quiescent vitamin A-rich cells to proliferative, fibrogenic and contractile myofibroblasts, which is termed "activation" or "trans-differentiation," [71]. Activated hepatic stellate cells possess numerous voltage-operated calcium channels [72]. Its activation is associated with the upregulation of L-type voltage-operated Ca^{2+} channels that mediate Ca^{2+} influx and cell contraction [73]. The change of intracellular Ca^{2+} concentration not only plays an important role in the activation of hepatic stellate cells but also plays a key role in the regression of fibrosis [74]. It has been found in medicine that the use of calcium blockers slows down liver fibrosis (Fig. **1**). Azelnidipine, a calcium blocker, can inhibit transforming growth factor beta-1 and angiotensin II-induced hepatic stellate cell activation *in vitro* and accelerate the regression of CCl4-induced liver fibrosis in mice [75].

An organism with an internal skeleton must accumulate calcium while maintaining body fluids at a well-regulated, constant calcium concentration. The major calcium regulatory mechanism of the body, the skeleton, in which calcium is deposited and removed by isoionic exchange, includes a process modulated by bone cells that in turn are subject to hormonal action and regulation. Ca^{2+} uptake and release by bone surfaces cause plasma calcium to be well regulated [76]. Therefore, prolonged chronic inflammation leads to a disturbance of calcium homeostasis *in vivo*, which may be one of the factors causing bone loss.

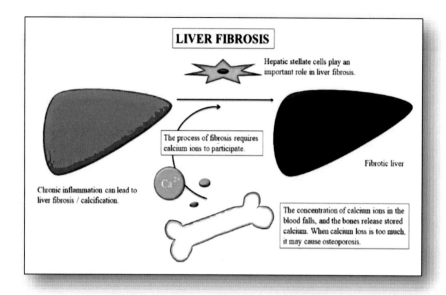

Fig. (1). Schematic diagram showing liver fibrosis due to extreme calcium loss.

Vitamin D

Vitamin D must be metabolized to 25(OH)D$_3$ in the liver and subsequently to 1,25(OH)$_2$D$_3$ in the kidney to produce its physiological actions [77]. Then, 1,25(OH)$_2$D$_3$ enhances bone mineralization through its effects to promote calcium and phosphate absorption [78]. Therefore, the disruption of vitamin D metabolic sequence or signaling system for 1,25(OH)$_2$D$_3$ results in several bone and calcium metabolism disorders [79].

Vitamin D through the vitamin D receptors (VDRs) plays a key role in mineral ion homeostasis [80]. VDRs are involved in expression in major cell populations of innate and adaptive immune responses. Dendritic cells and macrophages can produce 1,25(OH)$_2$D$_3$ within the microenvironment. This active form of vitamin D can inhibit immune cell proliferation, expand regulatory T cells, promote an anti-inflammatory cytokine profile, enhance glucocorticoid actions, and inhibit hepatic stellate cells [81]. It has abundant VDR expression in hepatic stellate cells. Through VDR signaling, it can inhibit the expression of fibrotic genes and the proliferation of hepatic stellate cells [82, 83]. In a study by Seydel *et al.*, LX-2 cells (one of the human hepatic stellate cell lines) and primary human hepatic stellate cells were treated with vitamin D2 (6~10 M) and free fatty acids at different concentrations (0.25 mM, 0.5 mM, and 1 mM) for 24 hours. The results showed that vitamin D2 can reduce the inflammatory and pro-fibrotic activity of hepatic stellate cells [84]. In addition, another study by Reiter *et al.* also showed that vitamin D3 can inhibit the hepatic stellate cell activation and proliferation in vitro, and can improve inflammatory liver damage in the ATP-binding cassette transporter b4 (-/-)-mice model by vitamin D3 [85].

Vitamin D deficiency is often associated with poor prognosis in chronic liver disease and osteoporosis. The prolonged chronic inflammation leads to a disturbance of calcium homeostasis [86 - 90].

CONCLUSION

It has been revealed that whether it is an autoimmune disease, metabolic syndrome, or hepatitis caused by viral infections, long-term inflammation of the liver promotes the occurrence of liver fibrosis. The process of fibrosis requires the participation of calcium ions. Osteoclasts release the calcium stored in the bone in order to balance the lost calcium ions. Therefore, liver fibrosis is often accompanied by bone loss. Patients with chronic hepatitis should also pay attention to bone health

REFERENCES

[1]   Iwasaki Y, Kazama JJ, Fukagawa M. Molecular abnormalities underlying bone fragility in chronic kidney disease. BioMed Res Int 2017; 1-11.
        [http://dx.doi.org/10.1155/2017/3485785] [PMID: 28421193]

[2]   Jean G, Souberbielle J, Chazot C. Vitamin D in chronic kidney disease and dialysis patients. Nutrients 2017; 9(4): 328.
        [http://dx.doi.org/10.3390/nu9040328] [PMID: 28346348]

[3]   Hoan NX, Tong HV, Song LH, Meyer CG, Velavan TP. Vitamin D deficiency and hepatitis viruses-associated liver diseases: A literature review. World J Gastroenterol 2018; 24(4): 445-60.
        [http://dx.doi.org/10.3748/wjg.v24.i4.445] [PMID: 29398866]

[4]   Holick MF, Siris ES, Binkley N, *et al.* Prevalence of Vitamin D inadequacy among postmenopausal North American women receiving osteoporosis therapy. J Clin Endocrinol Metab 2005; 90(6): 3215-24.
        [http://dx.doi.org/10.1210/jc.2004-2364] [PMID: 15797954]

[5]   Thomas MK, Lloyd-Jones DM, Thadhani RI, *et al.* Hypovitaminosis D in medical inpatients. N Engl J Med 1998; 338(12): 777-83.
        [http://dx.doi.org/10.1056/NEJM199803193381201] [PMID: 9504937]

[6]   Trefts E, Gannon M, Wasserman DH. The liver. Curr Biol 2017; 27(21): R1147-51.
        [http://dx.doi.org/10.1016/j.cub.2017.09.019] [PMID: 29112863]

[7]   Kubes P, Jenne C. Immune Responses in the Liver. Annu Rev Immunol 2018; 36(1): 247-77.
        [http://dx.doi.org/10.1146/annurev-immunol-051116-052415] [PMID: 29328785]

[8]   Luedde T, Kaplowitz N, Schwabe RF. Cell death and cell death responses in liver disease: Mechanisms and clinical relevance. Gastroenterology 2014; 147(4): 765-783.e4.
        [http://dx.doi.org/10.1053/j.gastro.2014.07.018] [PMID: 25046161]

[9]   Alshahrani F, Aljohani N. Vitamin D: deficiency, sufficiency and toxicity. Nutrients 2013; 5(9): 3605-16.
        [http://dx.doi.org/10.3390/nu5093605] [PMID: 24067388]

[10] Hoan NX, Khuyen N, Binh MT, *et al.* Association of vitamin D deficiency with hepatitis B virus : Related liver diseases. BMC Infect Dis 2016; 16(1): 507.
[http://dx.doi.org/10.1186/s12879-016-1836-0] [PMID: 27659316]

[11] Zhao X, Li J, Wang J, *et al.* Vitamin D serum level is associated with Child–Pugh score and metabolic enzyme imbalances, but not viral load in chronic hepatitis B patients. Medicine 2016; 95(27): e3926.
[http://dx.doi.org/10.1097/MD.0000000000003926] [PMID: 27399065]

[12] Petta S, Cammà C, Scazzone C, *et al.* Low vitamin D serum level is related to severe fibrosis and low responsiveness to interferon-based therapy in genotype 1 chronic hepatitis C. Hepatology 2010; 51(4): 1158-67.
[http://dx.doi.org/10.1002/hep.23489] [PMID: 20162613]

[13] Terrier B, Carrat F, Geri G, *et al.* Low 25-OH vitamin D serum levels correlate with severe fibrosis in HIV-HCV co-infected patients with chronic hepatitis. J Hepatol 2011; 55(4): 756-61.
[http://dx.doi.org/10.1016/j.jhep.2011.01.041] [PMID: 21334402]

[14] Iruzubieta P, Terán Á, Crespo J, Fábrega E. Vitamin D deficiency in chronic liver disease. World J Hepatol 2014; 6(12): 901-15.
[http://dx.doi.org/10.4254/wjh.v6.i12.901] [PMID: 25544877]

[15] Barchetta I, Cimini F, Cavallo M, Vitamin D. Vitamin D supplementation and non-alcoholic fatty liver disease: Present and future. Nutrients 2017; 9(9): 1015.
[http://dx.doi.org/10.3390/nu9091015] [PMID: 28906453]

[16] Xie X, Huang R, Li X, *et al.* Association between hepatitis B virus infection and risk of osteoporosis: A systematic review and meta-analysis. Medicine 2020; 99(16): e19719.
[http://dx.doi.org/10.1097/MD.0000000000019719] [PMID: 32311959]

[17] Trépo C, Chan HLY, Lok A. Hepatitis B virus infection. Lancet 2014; 384(9959): 2053-63.
[http://dx.doi.org/10.1016/S0140-6736(14)60220-8] [PMID: 24954675]

[18] Roggendorf M, Schlipköter U. Hepatitis C virus. Beitr Infusionsther 1991; 28: 13-21.
[PMID: 1725610]

[19] Chen YY, Fang WH, Wang CC, *et al.* Crosssectional assessment of bone mass density in adults with hepatitis B virus and hepatitis C virus infection. Sci Rep 2019; 9(1): 5069.
[http://dx.doi.org/10.1038/s41598-019-41674-4] [PMID: 30911051]

[20] Chen CH, Lin CL, Kao CH. Association between chronic hepatitis B virus infection and risk of osteoporosis. Medicine 2015; 94(50): e2276.
[http://dx.doi.org/10.1097/MD.0000000000002276] [PMID: 26683953]

[21] Farnik H, Bojunga J, Berger A, *et al.* Low vitamin D serum concentration is associated with high levels of hepatitis B virus replication in chronically infected patients. Hepatology 2013; 58(4): 1270-6.
[http://dx.doi.org/10.1002/hep.26488] [PMID: 23703797]

[22] Kong F, Zhang F, Liu X, *et al.* Calcium signaling in hepatitis B virus infection and its potential as a therapeutic target. Cell Commun Signal 2021; 19(1): 82.
[http://dx.doi.org/10.1186/s12964-021-00762-7] [PMID: 34362380]

[23] Mohamed AA, Abdo S, Said E, *et al.* Serum Vitamin D levels in chronic hepatitis B patients before and during treatment. Infect Disord Drug Targets 2021; 20(6): 840-7.
[http://dx.doi.org/10.2174/1871526519666191112112903] [PMID: 31721718]

[24] Lin JC, Hsieh TY, Wu CC, *et al.* Association between chronic hepatitis C virus infection and bone mineral density. Calcif Tissue Int 2012; 91(6): 423-9.
[http://dx.doi.org/10.1007/s00223-012-9653-y] [PMID: 23052227]

[25] Kanis JA, Cooper C, Rizzoli R, Reginster JY. Scientific advisory board of the european society for clinical and economic aspects of osteoporosis (ESCEO) and the committees of scientific advisors and national societies of the international osteoporosis foundation (IOF).European guidance for the

diagnosis and management of osteoporosis in postmenopausal women. Osteoporos Int 2019; 30(1): 3-44.
[http://dx.doi.org/10.1007/s00198-018-4704-5] [PMID: 30324412]

[26] Eastell R, Szulc P. Use of bone turnover markers in postmenopausal osteoporosis. Lancet Diabetes Endocrinol 2017; 5(11): 908-23.
[http://dx.doi.org/10.1016/S2213-8587(17)30184-5] [PMID: 28689768]

[27] Lai JC, Shoback DM, Zipperstein J, Lizaola B, Tseng S, Terrault NA. Bone mineral density, bone turnover, and systemic inflammation in non-cirrhotics with chronic hepatitis C. Dig Dis Sci 2015; 60(6): 1813-9.
[http://dx.doi.org/10.1007/s10620-014-3507-6] [PMID: 25563723]

[28] Rizzoli R. Nutritional aspects of bone health. Best Pract Res Clin Endocrinol Metab 2014; 28(6): 795-808.
[http://dx.doi.org/10.1016/j.beem.2014.08.003] [PMID: 25432353]

[29] Gutierrez J, Parikh N, Branch A. Classical and emerging roles of vitamin D in hepatitis C virus infection. Semin Liver Dis 2011; 31(4): 387-98.
[http://dx.doi.org/10.1055/s-0031-1297927] [PMID: 22189978]

[30] Cacopardo B, Camma C, Petta S, *et al.* Diagnostic and therapeutical role of vitamin D in chronic hepatitis C virus infection. Front Biosci 2012; E4(4): 1276-86.
[http://dx.doi.org/10.2741/e458] [PMID: 22201953]

[31] Selmi C, Generali E, Gershwin ME. Rheumatic manifestations in autoimmune liver disease. Rheum Dis Clin North Am 2018; 44(1): 65-87.
[http://dx.doi.org/10.1016/j.rdc.2017.09.008] [PMID: 29149928]

[32] Danford CJ, Trivedi HD, Papamichael K, Tapper EB, Bonder A. Osteoporosis in primary biliary cholangitis. World J Gastroenterol 2018; 24(31): 3513-20.
[http://dx.doi.org/10.3748/wjg.v24.i31.3513] [PMID: 30131657]

[33] Tsuneyama K, Baba H, Morimoto Y, Tsunematsu T, Ogawa H. Primary biliary cholangitis: Its pathological characteristics and immunopathological mechanisms. J Med Invest 2017; 64(1.2): 7-13.
[http://dx.doi.org/10.2152/jmi.64.7] [PMID: 28373632]

[34] Guañabens N, Parés A, Ros I, *et al.* Severity of cholestasis and advanced histological stage but not menopausal status are the major risk factors for osteoporosis in primary biliary cirrhosis. J Hepatol 2005; 42(4): 573-7.
[http://dx.doi.org/10.1016/j.jhep.2004.11.035] [PMID: 15763344]

[35] Parés A, Guañabens N. Osteoporosis in primary biliary cirrhosis: Pathogenesis and treatment. Clin Liver Dis 2008; 12(2): 407-24.
[http://dx.doi.org/10.1016/j.cld.2008.02.005] [PMID: 18456188]

[36] Lindor KD, Gershwin ME, Poupon R, Kaplan M, Bergasa NV, Heathcote EJ. Primary biliary cirrhosis. Hepatology 2009; 50(1): 291-308.
[http://dx.doi.org/10.1002/hep.22906] [PMID: 19554543]

[37] L Ng KV, Nguyễn LT. The role of vitamin d in primary biliary cirrhosis: Possible genetic and cell signaling mechanisms. Gastroenterol Res Pract 2013; 2013: 602321.
[PMID: 23589715]

[38] Wang Z, Peng C, Wang P, *et al.* Serum vitamin D level is related to disease progression in primary biliary cholangitis. Scand J Gastroenterol 2020; 55(11): 1333-40.
[http://dx.doi.org/10.1080/00365521.2020.1829030] [PMID: 33021858]

[39] McNally RJQ, James PW, Ducker S, James OFW. Seasonal variation in the patient diagnosis of primary biliary cirrhosis: Further evidence for an environmental component to etiology. Hepatology 2011; 54(6): 2099-103.
[http://dx.doi.org/10.1002/hep.24597] [PMID: 21826693]

[40] Gonzalez RS, Washington K. Primary biliary cholangitis and autoimmune hepatitis. Surg Pathol Clin 2018; 11(2): 329-49.
[http://dx.doi.org/10.1016/j.path.2018.02.010] [PMID: 29751878]

[41] Berg PA, Klein R. Autoimmune hepatitis and overlap syndrome: Diagnosis. Praxis 2002; 91: 1339-46.

[42] Schmidt T, Schmidt C, Strahl A, et al. A system to determine risk of osteoporosis in patients with autoimmune hepatitis. Clin Gastroenterol Hepatol 2020; 18(1): 226-233.e3.
[http://dx.doi.org/10.1016/j.cgh.2019.05.043] [PMID: 31163277]

[43] Abe K, Fujita M, Hayashi M, Takahashi A, Ohira H. Association of serum 25-hydroxyvitamin D levels with severe necroinflammatory activity and inflammatory cytokine production in type I autoimmune hepatitis. PLoS One 2020; 15(11): e0239481.
[http://dx.doi.org/10.1371/journal.pone.0239481] [PMID: 33151930]

[44] Ebadi M, Bhanji RA, Mazurak VC, et al. Severe vitamin D deficiency is a prognostic biomarker in autoimmune hepatitis. Aliment Pharmacol Ther 2019; 49(2): 173-82.
[http://dx.doi.org/10.1111/apt.15029] [PMID: 30484857]

[45] Rocco A, Compare D, Angrisani D, Sanduzzi Zamparelli M, Nardone G. Alcoholic disease: Liver and beyond. World J Gastroenterol 2014; 20(40): 14652-9.
[http://dx.doi.org/10.3748/wjg.v20.i40.14652] [PMID: 25356028]

[46] Cederbaum AI. Alcohol metabolism. Clin Liver Dis 2012; 16(4): 667-85.
[http://dx.doi.org/10.1016/j.cld.2012.08.002] [PMID: 23101976]

[47] Wosje KS, Kalkwarf HJ. Bone density in relation to alcohol intake among men and women in the United States. Osteoporos Int 2007; 18(3): 391-400.
[http://dx.doi.org/10.1007/s00198-006-0249-0] [PMID: 17091218]

[48] de Lorimier AA. Alcohol, wine, and health. Am J Surg 2000; 180(5): 357-61.
[http://dx.doi.org/10.1016/S0002-9610(00)00486-4] [PMID: 11137687]

[49] Feskanich D, Korrick SA, Greenspan SL, Rosen HN, Colditz GA. Moderate alcohol consumption and bone density among postmenopausal women. J Womens Health 1999; 8(1): 65-73.
[http://dx.doi.org/10.1089/jwh.1999.8.65] [PMID: 10094083]

[50] Laitinen K, Välimäki M. Alcohol and bone. Calcif Tissue Int 1991; 49(S1) (Suppl.): S70-3.
[http://dx.doi.org/10.1007/BF02555094] [PMID: 1933604]

[51] Tucker KL, Jugdaohsingh R, Powell JJ, et al. Effects of beer, wine, and liquor intakes on bone mineral density in older men and women. Am J Clin Nutr 2009; 89(4): 1188-96.
[http://dx.doi.org/10.3945/ajcn.2008.26765] [PMID: 19244365]

[52] May H, Murphy S, Khaw KT. Alcohol consumption and bone mineral density in older men. Gerontology 1995; 41(3): 152-8.
[http://dx.doi.org/10.1159/000213676] [PMID: 7601367]

[53] Hoyumpa AM. Mechanisms of vitamin deficiencies in alcoholism. Alcohol Clin Exp Res 1986; 10(6): 573-81.
[http://dx.doi.org/10.1111/j.1530-0277.1986.tb05147.x] [PMID: 3544907]

[54] Kizilgul M, Ozcelik O, Delibasi T. Bone health and vitamin D status in alcoholic liver disease. Indian J Gastroenterol 2016; 35(4): 253-9.
[http://dx.doi.org/10.1007/s12664-016-0652-1] [PMID: 27246833]

[55] López-Larramona G, Lucendo AJ, González-Delgado L. Alcoholic liver disease and changes in bone mineral density. Rev Esp Enferm Dig 2013; 105(10): 609-21.
[http://dx.doi.org/10.4321/S1130-01082013001000006] [PMID: 24641458]

[56] Eslam M, Sanyal AJ, George J, et al. MAFLD: A consensus-driven proposed nomenclature for metabolic associated fatty liver disease. Gastroenterology 2020; 158(7): 1999-2014.e1.
[http://dx.doi.org/10.1053/j.gastro.2019.11.312] [PMID: 32044314]

[57]   Zhou H, Ma C, Wang C, Gong L, Zhang Y, Li Y. Research progress in use of traditional Chinese medicine monomer for treatment of non-alcoholic fatty liver disease. Eur J Pharmacol 2021; 898: 173976.
[http://dx.doi.org/10.1016/j.ejphar.2021.173976] [PMID: 33639194]

[58]   Kim G, Kim KJ, Rhee Y, Lim SK. Significant liver fibrosis assessed using liver transient elastography is independently associated with low bone mineral density in patients with non-alcoholic fatty liver disease. PLoS One 2017; 12(7): e0182202.
[http://dx.doi.org/10.1371/journal.pone.0182202] [PMID: 28759632]

[59]   Pardee PE, Dunn W, Schwimmer JB. Non-alcoholic fatty liver disease is associated with low bone mineral density in obese children. Aliment Pharmacol Ther 2012; 35(2): 248-54.
[http://dx.doi.org/10.1111/j.1365-2036.2011.04924.x] [PMID: 22111971]

[60]   Sharifi N, Amani R, Hajiani E, Cheraghian B. Does vitamin D improve liver enzymes, oxidative stress, and inflammatory biomarkers in adults with non-alcoholic fatty liver disease? A randomized clinical trial. Endocrine 2014; 47(1): 70-80.
[http://dx.doi.org/10.1007/s12020-014-0336-5] [PMID: 24968737]

[61]   Wan B, Gao Y, Zheng Y, Chen R. Association between serum 25-hydroxy vitamin D level and metabolic associated fatty liver disease (MAFLD)—a population-based study. Endocr J 2021; 68(6): 631-7.
[http://dx.doi.org/10.1507/endocrj.EJ20-0758] [PMID: 33658438]

[62]   Guan Y, Xu Y, Su H, Sun X, Li Y, Wang T. Effect of serum vitamin D on metabolic associated fatty liver disease: A large population-based study. Scand J Gastroenterol 2022; 57(7): 862-71.
[http://dx.doi.org/10.1080/00365521.2022.2039284] [PMID: 35170370]

[63]   Yilmaz Y. Review article: Non-alcoholic fatty liver disease and osteoporosis : Clinical and molecular crosstalk. Aliment Pharmacol Ther 2012; 36(4): 345-52.
[http://dx.doi.org/10.1111/j.1365-2036.2012.05196.x] [PMID: 22730920]

[64]   Friedman SL. Liver fibrosis : From bench to bedside. J Hepatol 2003; 38 (1): 38-53.
[http://dx.doi.org/10.1016/S0168-8278(02)00429-4] [PMID: 12591185]

[65]   Bataller R, Brenner DA. Liver fibrosis. J Clin Invest 2005; 115(2): 209-18.
[http://dx.doi.org/10.1172/JCI24282] [PMID: 15690074]

[66]   Pellicoro A, Ramachandran P, Iredale JP, Fallowfield JA. Liver fibrosis and repair: Immune regulation of wound healing in a solid organ. Nat Rev Immunol 2014; 14(3): 181-94.
[http://dx.doi.org/10.1038/nri3623] [PMID: 24566915]

[67]   Higashi T, Friedman SL, Hoshida Y. Hepatic stellate cells as key target in liver fibrosis. Adv Drug Deliv Rev 2017; 121: 27-42.
[http://dx.doi.org/10.1016/j.addr.2017.05.007] [PMID: 28506744]

[68]   Wallace M, Mann D, Friedman S. Emerging and disease-specific mechanisms of hepatic stellate cell activation. Semin Liver Dis 2015; 35(2): 107-18.
[http://dx.doi.org/10.1055/s-0035-1550060] [PMID: 25974897]

[69]   Canbay A, Friedman S, Gores GJ. Apoptosis: The nexus of liver injury and fibrosis. Hepatology 2004; 39(2): 273-8.
[http://dx.doi.org/10.1002/hep.20051] [PMID: 14767974]

[70]   Koyama Y, Brenner DA. Liver inflammation and fibrosis. J Clin Invest 2017; 127(1): 55-64.
[http://dx.doi.org/10.1172/JCI88881] [PMID: 28045404]

[71]   Friedman SL. Molecular regulation of hepatic fibrosis, an integrated cellular response to tissue injury. J Biol Chem 2000; 275(4): 2247-50.
[http://dx.doi.org/10.1074/jbc.275.4.2247] [PMID: 10644669]

[72]   Bataller R, Nicolás JM, Ginès P, *et al.* Contraction of human hepatic stellate cells activated in culture:

A role for voltage-operated calcium channels. J Hepatol 1998; 29(3): 398-408.
[http://dx.doi.org/10.1016/S0168-8278(98)80057-3] [PMID: 9764986]

[73]   Bataller R, Gasull X, Ginès P, *et al.* *In vitro and in vivo* activation of rat hepatic stellate cells results in de novo expression of L-type voltage-operated calcium channels. Hepatology 2001; 33(4): 956-62.
[http://dx.doi.org/10.1053/jhep.2001.23500] [PMID: 11283860]

[74]   Chen CC, Hsu LW, Chen KD, Chiu KW, Chen CL, Huang KT. Emerging roles of calcium signaling in the development of non-alcoholic fatty liver disease. Int J Mol Sci 2021; 23(1): 256.
[http://dx.doi.org/10.3390/ijms23010256] [PMID: 35008682]

[75]   Ohyama T, Sato K, Kishimoto K, *et al.* Azelnidipine is a calcium blocker that attenuates liver fibrosis and may increase antioxidant defence. Br J Pharmacol 2012; 165(4b): 1173-87.
[http://dx.doi.org/10.1111/j.1476-5381.2011.01599.x] [PMID: 21790536]

[76]   Bronner F. Extracellular and intracellular regulation of calcium homeostasis. ScientiWorJ 2001; 1: 919-25.
[http://dx.doi.org/10.1100/tsw.2001.489] [PMID: 12805727]

[77]   DeLuca HF. Vitamin D-dependent calcium transport. Soc Gen Physiol Ser 1985; 39: 159-76.
[PMID: 2984778]

[78]   Yoshida T, Stern PH. How vitamin D works on bone. Endocrinol Metab Clin North Am 2012; 41(3): 557-69.
[http://dx.doi.org/10.1016/j.ecl.2012.04.003] [PMID: 22877429]

[79]   DeLUCA HF. Vitamin D endocrinology. Ann Intern Med 1976; 85(3): 367-77.
[http://dx.doi.org/10.7326/0003-4819-85-3-367] [PMID: 183579]

[80]   Zúñiga S, Firrincieli D, Housset C, Chignard N. Vitamin D and the vitamin D receptor in liver pathophysiology. Clin Res Hepatol Gastroenterol 2011; 35(4): 295-302.
[http://dx.doi.org/10.1016/j.clinre.2011.02.003] [PMID: 21440524]

[81]   Czaja AJ, Montano-Loza AJ. Evolving role of vitamin D in immune-mediated disease and its implications in autoimmune hepatitis. Dig Dis Sci 2019; 64(2): 324-44.
[http://dx.doi.org/10.1007/s10620-018-5351-6] [PMID: 30370494]

[82]   Ding N, Yu RT, Subramaniam N, *et al.* A vitamin D receptor/SMAD genomic circuit gates hepatic fibrotic response. Cell 2013; 153(3): 601-13.
[http://dx.doi.org/10.1016/j.cell.2013.03.028] [PMID: 23622244]

[83]   Abramovitch S, Dahan-Bachar L, Sharvit E, *et al.* Vitamin D inhibits proliferation and profibrotic marker expression in hepatic stellate cells and decreases thioacetamide-induced liver fibrosis in rats. Gut 2011; 60(12): 1728-37.
[http://dx.doi.org/10.1136/gut.2010.234666] [PMID: 21816960]

[84]   Seydel S, Beilfuss A, Kahraman A, *et al.* Vitamin D ameliorates stress ligand expression elicited by free fatty acids in the hepatic stellate cell line LX-2. Turk J Gastroenterol 2011; 22(4): 400-7.
[http://dx.doi.org/10.4318/tjg.2011.0254] [PMID: 21948571]

[85]   Reiter FP, Hohenester S, Nagel JM, *et al.* 1,25-(OH)2-vitamin D3 prevents activation of hepatic stellate cells *in vitro* and ameliorates inflammatory liver damage but not fibrosis in the Abcb4−/− model. Biochem Biophys Res Commun 2015; 459(2): 227-33.
[http://dx.doi.org/10.1016/j.bbrc.2015.02.074] [PMID: 25712522]

[86]   Paternostro R, Wagner D, Reiberger T, *et al.* Low 25-OH-vitamin D levels reflect hepatic dysfunction and are associated with mortality in patients with liver cirrhosis. Wien Klin Wochenschr 2017; 129(1-2): 8-15.
[http://dx.doi.org/10.1007/s00508-016-1127-1] [PMID: 27888359]

[87]   Finkelmeier F, Kronenberger B, Zeuzem S, Piiper A, Waidmann O. Low 25-Hydroxyvitamin D levels are associated with infections and mortality in patients with cirrhosis. PLoS One 2015; 10(6): e0132119.

[http://dx.doi.org/10.1371/journal.pone.0132119] [PMID: 26121590]

[88]   Stokes CS, Krawczyk M, Reichel C, Lammert F, Grünhage F. Vitamin D deficiency is associated with mortality in patients with advanced liver cirrhosis. Eur J Clin Invest 2014; 44(2): 176-83.
[http://dx.doi.org/10.1111/eci.12205] [PMID: 24236541]

[89]   Wang X, Li W, Zhang Y, Yang Y, Qin G. Association between vitamin D and non-alcoholic fatty liver disease/non-alcoholic steatohepatitis: results from a meta-analysis. Int J Clin Exp Med 2015; 8(10): 17221-34.
[PMID: 26770315]

[90]   Putz-Bankuti C, Pilz S, Stojakovic T, *et al.* Association of 25-hydroxyvitamin D levels with liver dysfunction and mortality in chronic liver disease. Liver Int 2012; 32(5): 845-51.
[http://dx.doi.org/10.1111/j.1478-3231.2011.02735.x] [PMID: 22222013]

CHAPTER 2

Detection of Knee Osteoarthritis using Artificial Intelligence

Pongphak Thongpat[1], Napat Pongsakonpruttikul[1] and Chayanin Angthong[1,*]

[1] *Facutly of Medicine, King Mongkut's Institute of Technology Ladkrabang (KMITL), Bangkok, Thailand*

Abstract: Knee osteoarthritis (KOA) is a common degenerative joint disease that results in disability due to joint dysfunction and pain. Almost one-fifth of early KOA cases are missed during the routine practice resulting in the progression of the disease. This narrative review aimed to explore and analyze various literatures that proposed Convoluted Neural Network (CNN) model in detecting KOA and its severity based on Kellgren Lawrence grading classification. At first, 221 publications were retrieved using the search term "artificial intelligence" and Knee osteoarthritis". Only studies that used CNN and radiographic images were included in this study in which only 14 studies fitted our inclusion criteria. Each paper was thoroughly investigated for the input data and CNN model adopted as well as the performance and limitation of that study. Lastly, the conclusion was made and discussed using these results. Object detection and Classification models were among the most popular techniques adopted. Our results showed that object detection models were overall superior regarding the accuracy in the detection of KOA and its severity. The application of CNN for the detection of KOA from radiographic images has shown great promise where each technique has its own advantage. In the foreseeable future, the combination of object detection and classification detection may provide excellent potential as a merit tool to help orthopedists and related physicians for the proper diagnosis and treatment of KOA.

Keywords: Artificial intelligence, Knee osteoarthritis, Radiographic image.

INTRODUCTION

Knee osteoarthritis (KOA) is a degenerative joint disease that causes pain and restricted range of motion which may lead to a decline in the quality of life [1 - 3]. It is a chronic disorder typically known as a result of wear and tear processes leading to progressive destruction of the articular cartilage and, ultimately, functional disability [4]. The symptom of knee pain during weight-bearing activities is one of the earliest signs [5]. If left untreated, it could progress to

----
[*] **Corresponding author Chayanin Angthong:** Facutly of Medicine, King Mongkut's Institute of Technology Ladkrabang (KMITL), Bangkok, Thailand; Tel: +662-329-8085; E-mail: Chayanin.an@kmitl.ac.th

disability due to the decrease in range of motion (ROM) of the knee and the inability to walk. The current definite mainstay treatment for advanced-stage KOA is knee joint replacement which is costly and places a huge burden on the overall healthcare cost [6, 7]. With this, the focus of treatment has been shifted towards prevention and treatment during the early stage [6, 7]. Although early intervention can prevent further degeneration, up to 15% of early KOA are left undetected during routine practice [8, 9]. Due to the recent emergence of Artificial Intelligence (AI), there has been a growing trend in its application in tackling medical problems. The detection of KOA with the adoption of AI may help physicians in detecting and localizing pathological lesions of the knee.

AI was first defined as the ability of a machine to learn and solve problems. With its complex algorithm-based processing, it allows machines to learn by using hidden layers (decision tree) making it applicable in many fields of medicine [1]. A convolutional neural network (CNN) or deep learning system is a sophisticated technique that mimics the human nervous system by including many layers of processing. These layers include the input layers, hidden layers and the output layers, which allow the identification of complex patterns in comparison with traditional machine learning techniques [10 - 13]. Due to CNN's fast processing ability, it can be used for real-time detection of the desired object in an image or video, a technique known as Computer vision. Many previous studies have demonstrated the usefulness of CNN in aiding the diagnosis of many diseases from various diagnostic investigations, including histological imaging, radiographic imaging and magnetic resonance imaging (MRI). The detection of pathologic lesions in KOA is a prime example of how AI could assist physicians [5, 10 - 22].

There has been much research conducted on machine learning in the past that aims at assisting physicians in the diagnosis of diseases. Algorithm-based machine learning using patient information such as age, patient history, risk factors, and predisposing illness can help predict the outcome of the disease [12]. Currently, there has been growing popularity in the field of computer vision to detect pathological lesions shown in radiography. The AI-assisted methods have been increasingly implemented in diagnosing and treating KOA. This review aims to present the potential of AI, as well as its limitations, in the detection of KOA using radiographic imaging.

MATERIAL AND METHODS

First, we retrieved a total of 221 studies from PubMed and Google Scholar published between 2000 and 2021. The search keywords used were "artificial intelligence and knee osteoarthritis". Then further screening was performed, where articles that were published in the English language, had full text, contained keywords of radiographic images and adopted CNN were included for this review. Exclusion criteria were articles that were not written in the English language, published before the year 2000 and studies that were conducted with MRI or CT images and used shallow machine learning algorithms. Duplicates were also excluded. Finally, only 14 publications were selected for this narrative review. The workflow of the identification of studies is shown in Fig. (**1**).

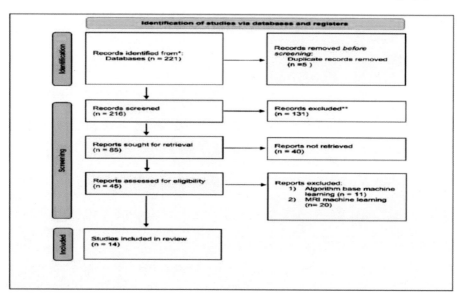

Fig. (1). Identification of studies.

The learning algorithm, model validation method, results and limitations of each individual study were explored. Then, these parameters were compared and analyzed. Lastly, the result of our analysis was discussed and concluded.

DETECTION OF KNEE OSTEOARTHRITIS BY AI

Detection of KOA using AI can be helpful for medical practitioners during their daily practices. However, there are challenges associated with training the AI. Even though many individuals might have similar body structures, no two people are exactly identical, and this is certainly true for the structure of the knee [5]. In building the basis for AI training, consistency of information is critical. If the information is not consistent, AI would need a greater amount of input information to provide a satisfactory result in terms of detection performance. In KOA radiography, the pathological presentations are osteophytes, subchondral bone sclerosis, and bone structure which may display great variations among different individuals. This may pose a great hurdle in the training of the deep learning model [22]. For this reason, the major pain point is the variety of macro-structural information from radiographic images that AI needs to be able to differentiate [17 - 20]. Most of the studies that have developed AI models mainly focus on the macro-structural bio-information analysis and detect KOA based on the Kellgren-Lawrence classification for severity grading in radiographic images [22].

According to our review, two main deep learning methods have been proposed for the detection of KOA: "object detection" and "classification". Classification uses semi-supervised learning to group the common KOA grading based on the ground truth, while object detection uses fully supervised learning for AI to detect a specific location of the lesion based on the labeling of the region of interest of the pathological site [1, 10 - 21]. Object detection has a sensitivity range of 65% to 78% and a specificity range of 87% to 94% [16 - 21]. On the other hand, classification has a sensitivity range of 66.7% to 100%, a specificity range of 74.6% to 100%, an accuracy range of 66.71% to 95% and a receiver operating characteristic (ROC) range of 0.79 to 0.93 [1, 10 - 15]. The results are variable and discussed below.

GRADING OF KOA: KELLGREN AND LAWRENCE CLASSIFICATION AND ITS SHORTCOMINGS

The Kellgren and Lawrence system for the classification of osteoarthritis (KL grading) is one of the most standardized KOA radiographic image grading systems [23]. The grading is based on the pathomorphological changes in KOA, such as narrowing of the joint space, osteophytes, and subchondral bone sclerosis (Fig. **2**, Table **1**). Even though it is widely adopted, its grading is not perfect and has some shortcomings. First, KL grading is very subjective as it relies heavily on the physician's experience and observation skills. With this, it would not be surprising that small osteophyte lesions can easily be missed by an untrained eye. This is especially true in the lower KL gradings, such as KL1 and KL2, in which the definitions are very similar that makes distinguishing the two groups difficult and prone to misinterpretation [11, 14, 15]. Secondly, there is an ambiguity in the description in each class as there is no set of standards in the description of each lesion [24, 25]. For example, there is no exact measurement that would describe the joint as "narrowing". Furthermore, one study conducted an intra-observer analysis of KL among experienced observers and concluded a lack in reproducibility and gave only superficial agreement among observers using Krippendorff's alpha coefficient [26]. In addition, the Kappa coefficient for KL grading varies from one research study to another [27].

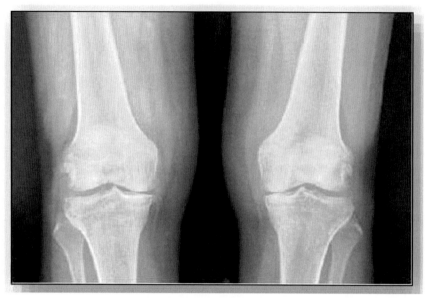

Fig. (2). Anteroposterior radiograph demonstrating knee osteoarthritis with KL grade 3.

Table 1. Kellgren-Lawrence classification of knee osteoarthritis [25, 27].

KL 0	Definite absence of x-ray changes of osteoarthritis.
KL 1	Doubtful joint space narrowing and possible osteophytic lipping.
KL 2	Definite osteophytes and possible joint space narrowing.
KL 3	Moderate multiple osteophytes, definite narrowing of joint space and some sclerosis and possible deformity of bone ends.
KL 4	Large osteophytes, marked narrowing of joint space, severe sclerosis and definite deformity of bone ends.

The difficulty in classifying KOA using KL grading can affect the result of AI performance [1, 10 - 17]. This is because the input data must first be correctly classified into different groups prior to feeding them to the model for training. However, as mentioned, the task is highly operator-dependent, and the ground truth made might be lacking in the accuracy and consistency of lesion labeling. As a result, AI might learn using this misinterpreted input resulting in an overfitting problem. This will likely lower the accuracy, sensitivity, and specificity of AI itself in real life situations. There are many approaches to solve this problem; one of the examples is grouping the KL grading into broader classification such as normal, mild, moderate, and severe. One article by Tiulpin *et al.* has bypassed this problem by grading KOA as normal or osteoarthritis. Another approach to this is to use two experienced radiologists to grade KOA radiography to increase the accuracy of the ground truth for AI to be trained on [19, 20].

CONVOLUTIONAL NEURAL NETWORK: CLASSIFICATION MODEL

The classification detection model (Fig. **3A**, Table **2**) uses the "data pooling" of the fine details of images for learning and classifying them into a class system, under semi-unsupervised learning. The class system is sorted by the operator in the grouping of the data in each grading. The pathological lesion localization involves AI "seeing" the differences between each group and highlighting what it sees. Then, the deep learning model would draw a heat map around one or more objects on the image that represent the pathological site. The color of the heat map will be intensified at the area of interest and display the group it belongs to based on the ground truth that AI is trained upon. The result of the CNN classification model can be shown as the probability of the input being in the represented class [1, 10, 11]. This method of classification has the advantage of reducing human error during the process of training [10, 11]. It reduces human error and can detect new information that humans may overlook in the macro biomarker of the disease *via* computer vision. The performance of the classification model in CNN can increase its accuracy and precision by increasing the amount of data it has been trained with [11].

Furthermore, the CNN-based classification detection model will present the heat map that helps the operator indicate the location where AI is looking. It will benefit the operator who operates the machine in the diagnosis of the disease using KOA radiography.

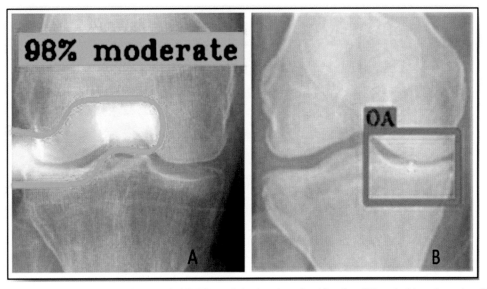

Fig. (3). Convolutional neural network (CNN) models showing classification (**A**) and object detection (**B**). Images courtesy of the Osteoarthritis Initiative (OAI).

Table 2. Summary of previous AI studies on knee osteoarthritis.

Author	Year	Learning Algorithm	Validation	Results	Limitation
Joseph Antony	2016	CaffeNet	Confusion matrix	Sensitivity 65% and specificity 87%	The KL grading doesn't have clear definition for KL.
Joseph Antony	2017	Elastic Net	Confusion matrix	Mean ROC is 87%	Actual image of Knee OA is used
Berk Norman	2018	DenseNets	Confusion matrix	Sensitivity 77.2%, specificity 91.5%	The ground truth using KL grading is subjective
Aleksei Tiulpin	2018	Deep Siamese convolutional neural network	Confusion matrix	66.71% accuracy 0.93 ROC curve	Both KL1 and KL2 have low specificity
Jaynal Abedin	2019	Elastic Net	Root mean square	Regression model is 0.97, random forest model is 0.94	High subjectivity between radiologists in KL grading
AbdelbassetBrahim	2019	ResNet	Naïve Bayes classifiers and Leave-One-Out cross validation.	82.98% accuracy, 87.15% sensitivity, 80.65% specificity	Low sensitivity and specificity in detecting early KOA
Aleksei Tiulpin	2019	Resnext50-32xd	Cross-validation comparing with OAI data	0.79 ROC curve, Average Precision 0.68	AI can only be used in standard radiographic image, only rely on KL grading, ignore symptoms of KOA, and use imputation in training AI.
Kevin Leung	2020	ResNet34	Sevenfold cross-validation	AUC of 0.87	Limited data set at 780 compared to OAI at 3000. The result is taken as binary.
Bin Liu	2020	Faster R-CNN	Confusion matrix	Average precision 82%, sensitivity 78%, specificity 94%	The quality of the annotation of the marking area has a great influence on the accuracy.

(Table 2) cont.....

Author	Year	Learning Algorithm	Validation	Results	Limitation
Paul H. Yi	2020	ResNet18 ResNet152	Confusion matrix	95% accuracy, 100% sensitivity, 100% specificity	A small sample size could possibly result in overfitting
Simon Olsson	2021	ResNet	Confusion matrix	Mean ROC curve 0.92, mean sensitivity 92%, mean specificity 74.6%.	Many Deep learning models were implemented. KL grading suffers from ambiguity due to inter-observer reliability.
Albert Swiecicki	2021	VGG16	Confusion matrix	Multi-class accuracy of 71.90% PA view, 61.18% LAT view Kappa coefficient of 0.769	The KL grading is used for measurement of severity of OA. There is a difference between the CNN and radiologist reading.
Mohammed Bany Muhammad	2021	MobileNet v1	Confusion matrix	Mean sensitivity is 87%	A low performance in classifying KL1.

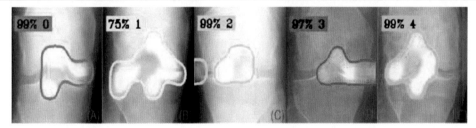

Fig. (4). AI detection of knee osteoarthritis using Kellgren Lawrence classification. (**A**) KL0 with 99% confidence, normal knee. (**B**) KL1 75% confidence, doubtful joint space narrowing and osteophyte. (**C**) KL2 99% confidence, definite joint space narrowing with possible osteophyte. (**D**) KL3 97% confidence, definite joint space narrowing with multiple osteophytic lesions, and possible deformity of bone architecture. (**E**) KL4 99% confidence, Marked joint space narrowing with subchondral bone sclerosis, definite deformity of the bone end.

CONVOLUTIONAL NEURAL NETWORK: OBJECT DETECTION MODEL

The use of CNN with an object detection model (Fig. **3B**, Table **2**) involves two tasks: the operator drawing a bounding box around the area of interest and assigning class labeling. The operator needs to identify and mark the location of the pathology for CNN to be able to detect its landmark. The CNN operates on supervised learning, with a more specific marking of the pathologic location on the image, which increases the performance of CNN. Object detection works by identifying the operator-dependent marked location on the image while verifying pixels to provide the result [8]. It is used predominantly to identify many structures in an image simultaneously and can be used in KOA radiography [10]. The most common approach that has been taken in object detection involves the segmentation of the joint space and focuses on the medial part of the knee [23].

DISCUSSION

Over 4% of the world population or 250 million people worldwide are affected by Osteoarthritis (OA) [28]. By 2010, approximately 17 million years lost to disability was due to OA with roughly 80% being caused by KOA alone [28]. The current gold standard in the diagnosis of KOA is the combination of clinical presentation and radiographic image. AI can assist physicians in detecting and classifying the severity of KOA (Fig. **4**). Especially with the advancement in the application of deep learning in the field of computer vision, it can be used for image detection by adapting its function for the detection of medical images. With the ongoing increase in the collection of sample size, it would be beneficial for CNN in terms of its accuracy and other performance parameters. To increase the performance of the CNN, each factor used in the CNN training is needed to fine-tune the model. Aspects that warrant further investigation are the KL grading criteria, the models of CNN detection and the site/pattern of detection, and the source of data for running CNN experiments.

The KL grading classification for KOA is used widely for grading KOA on plain radiography, but it is far from perfect [25]. Due to the differing definitions of an osteophyte and the subjectivity associated with the detection of osteophytes, the grading of KOA is found challenging. Most articles in this review have stated that KL grading is based on the subjective assessment of the operator, especially in KL1 and KL2. For KL0, KL3, and KL4, the pathological site is very well-defined, and AI can detect it with high accuracy [12 - 21]. Yi *et al.* suggested an alternative approach based on grading of severity to resolve this problem. The severity is graded as normal, mild, moderate, and severe based on the medical treatment the patient is expected to receive [22]. As a result, grouping the problematic KL1 and KL2 grades together increases the accuracy of the detection [22]. Another suggested approach is to use two experienced radiologists to grade KOA, creating intra- and inter-observer reproducibility. This would reduce individual subjectivity and create a more standardized dataset [17].

In the case of object detection for CNN AI training, it is operator-dependent. The operator needs to mark and grade the pathological site for training AI. Therefore, fatigability comes into play [15]. However, in AI training, an abundance of annotated medical images is much needed. Taking into consideration that KOA involves biological imaging, in which there is no one common structure, this creates a verity of the ground truth, lowering the accuracy of AI [18, 19].

Comparing object detection and classification models, object detection provides a more superior result in terms of accuracy, whereas classification is associated with more practical detection that can be used in clinics, involving so-called "heat maps". Each detection model is associated with superiority in its own way, determined by the objective of each article.

Furthermore, more research needs to be performed to improve the accuracy of AI in the detection of KOA by combining all the methods discussed above, including object detection and classification, as well as moving from a KL classification to a severity classification. Future research should focus on combining object detection and classification models and creating a 2-layer CNN to improve AI performance. All of the previous research have only focused on AI in the overall detection of the knee capsule, but the most common pathological site of KOA is the medial side of the knee. Focusing on the medial part of the knee should increase the AI performance. Lastly, for all reviewed articles, datasets of KOA radiographic images have been derived from two public resources which are the OAI (Osteoarthritis Initiative) and MOST (Multicenter Osteoarthritis Study). OAI is a multicentric, longitudinal, prospective observational study of KOA sponsored by the US National Institutes of Health (NIH). It is a private and public partnership that aims to provide a publicly accessible database of knee OA. It contains biomarkers and radiographic images collected since 2014 [29]. As for MOST, it is also a longitudinal, prospective, observational study of KOA conducted by two research centers. It seeks to identify biomechanical factors, bone and joint structural factors and nutritional factors that influence KOA [30]. However, at the moment of this review, MOST has been shut down due to inadequate funding. From our results, it has been revealed that articles that have chosen OAI as their dataset of choice in the development of the CNN model, show a lower performance in regard to sensitivity, specificity, accuracy, and ROC curve as compared to the results obtained when the MOST and OAI datasets are combined. The solution to this prior research would be to obtain more radiographic images from other sources

CONCLUSION

Convoluted neural networks should be further investigated for its role in detecting KOA on radiographic images. In terms of clinical usage, it could potentially aid physicians not only in the diagnosis but also in assessing the severity of KOA. This allows early detection of KOA in the initial stage and permits physicians to treat patients according to the severity of their disease. Overall, CNN may be able to assist the physicians in determining the pathologic site, the possible severity and viable treatment for KOA. In the foreseeable future, AI with a combination of object detection and classification detection may provide excellent potential as a merit tool to help orthopedists and related physicians in the proper diagnosis and treatment of KOA.

REFERENCES

[1] Abedin J, Antony J, McGuinness K, *et al.* Predicting knee osteoarthritis severity: Comparative modeling based on patient's data and plain X-ray images. Sci Rep 2019; 9(1): 5761.
[http://dx.doi.org/10.1038/s41598-019-42215-9] [PMID: 30962509]

[2] Kanamoto T, Mae T, Yokoyama T, Tanaka H, Ebina K, Nakata K. Significance and definition of early knee osteoarthritis. Ann Joint 2020; 5: 4.
[http://dx.doi.org/10.21037/aoj.2019.09.02]

[3] Vaishya R, Pariyo GB, Agarwal AK, Vijay V. Non-operative management of osteoarthritis of the knee joint. J Clin Orthop Trauma 2016; 7(3): 170-6.
[http://dx.doi.org/10.1016/j.jcot.2016.05.005] [PMID: 27489412]

[4] Hsu H, Siwiec R. Knee Osteoarthritis. StatPearls 2022. Available from: https://www.ncbi.nlm.nih.gov/books/NBK507884/ (cited 2022 Sep 20)

[5] Bliddal H, Leeds AR, Stigsgaard L, Astrup A, Christensen R. Weight loss as treatment for knee osteoarthritis symptoms in obese patients: 1-year results from a randomised controlled trial. Ann Rheum Dis 2011; 70(10): 1798-803.
[http://dx.doi.org/10.1136/ard.2010.142018] [PMID: 21821622]

[6] Cui A, Li H, Wang D, Zhong J, Chen Y, Lu H. Global, regional prevalence, incidence and risk factors of knee osteoarthritis in population-based studies. EClinicalMedicine 2020; 29-30: 100587.
[http://dx.doi.org/10.1016/j.eclinm.2020.100587] [PMID: 34505846]

[7] Glyn-Jones S, Palmer AJR, Agricola R, *et al.* Osteoarthritis. Lancet 2015; 386(9991): 376-87.
[http://dx.doi.org/10.1016/S0140-6736(14)60802-3] [PMID: 25748615]

[8] Pongsakonpruttikul N, Angthong C, Kittichai V, *et al.* Artificial intelligence assistance in radiographic detection and classification of knee osteoarthritis and its severity: A cross-sectional diagnostic study. Eur Rev Med Pharmacol Sci 2022; 26(5): 1549-58.
[PMID: 35302199]

[9] Chaisson CE, Gale DR, Gale E, Kazis L, Skinner K, Felson DT. Detecting radiographic knee osteoarthritis: what combination of views is optimal? Rheumatology 2000; 39(11): 1218-21.
[http://dx.doi.org/10.1093/rheumatology/39.11.1218] [PMID: 11085800]

[10] Antony J, McGuinness K, Moran K, O'Connor NE. Automatic detection of knee joints and quantification of knee osteoarthritis severity using convolutional neural networks. International conference on machine learning and data mining in pattern recognition. 376-90.
[http://dx.doi.org/10.1007/978-3-319-62416-7_27]

[11] Antony J, McGuinness K, O'Connor NE, Moran K. Quantifying radiographic knee osteoarthritis severity using deep convolutional neural networks. 2016 23rd International Conference on Pattern Recognition (ICPR),. 04-08 December, Cancun, Mexico, 2016, pp. 1195-1200.
[http://dx.doi.org/10.1109/ICPR.2016.7899799]

[12] Bany Muhammad M, Yeasin M. Interpretable and parameter optimized ensemble model for knee

osteoarthritis assessment using radiographs. Sci Rep 2021; 11(1): 14348.
[http://dx.doi.org/10.1038/s41598-021-93851-z] [PMID: 34253839]

[13] Brahim A, Jennane R, Riad R, *et al.* A decision support tool for early detection of knee OsteoArthritis using X-ray imaging and machine learning: Data from the OsteoArthritis Initiative. Comput Med Imaging Graph 2019; 73: 11-8.
[http://dx.doi.org/10.1016/j.compmedimag.2019.01.007] [PMID: 30784984]

[14] Leung K, Zhang B, Tan J, *et al.* Prediction of total knee replacement and diagnosis of osteoarthritis by using deep learning on knee radiographs: Data from the osteoarthritis initiative. Radiology 2020; 296(3): 584-93.
[http://dx.doi.org/10.1148/radiol.2020192091] [PMID: 32573386]

[15] Liu B, Luo J, Huang H. Toward automatic quantification of knee osteoarthritis severity using improved Faster R-CNN. Int J CARS 2020; 15(3): 457-66.
[http://dx.doi.org/10.1007/s11548-019-02096-9] [PMID: 31938993]

[16] Norman B, Pedoia V, Noworolski A, Link TM, Majumdar S. Applying densely connected convolutional neural networks for staging osteoarthritis severity from plain radiographs. J Digit Imaging 2019; 32(3): 471-7.
[http://dx.doi.org/10.1007/s10278-018-0098-3] [PMID: 30306418]

[17] Olsson S, Akbarian E, Lind A, Razavian AS, Gordon M. Automating classification of osteoarthritis according to Kellgren-Lawrence in the knee using deep learning in an unfiltered adult population. BMC Musculoskelet Disord 2021; 22(1): 844.
[http://dx.doi.org/10.1186/s12891-021-04722-7] [PMID: 34600505]

[18] Swiecicki A, Li N, O'Donnell J, *et al.* Deep learning-based algorithm for assessment of knee osteoarthritis severity in radiographs matches performance of radiologists. Comput Biol Med 2021; 133: 104334.
[http://dx.doi.org/10.1016/j.compbiomed.2021.104334] [PMID: 33823398]

[19] Tiulpin A, Klein S, Bierma-Zeinstra SMA, *et al.* Multimodal machine learning-based knee osteoarthritis progression prediction from plain radiographs and clinical data. Sci Rep 2019; 9(1): 20038.
[http://dx.doi.org/10.1038/s41598-019-56527-3] [PMID: 31882803]

[20] Tiulpin A, Thevenot J, Rahtu E, Lehenkari P, Saarakkala S. Automatic knee osteoarthritis diagnosis from plain radiographs: A deep learning-based approach. Sci Rep 2018; 8(1): 1727.
[http://dx.doi.org/10.1038/s41598-018-20132-7] [PMID: 29379060]

[21] Wahyuningrum RT, Purnama IKE, Verkerke GJ, van Ooijen PMA, Purnomo MH. A novel method for determining the Femoral-Tibial Angle of Knee Osteoarthritis on X-ray radiographs: data from the Osteoarthritis Initiative. Heliyon 2020; 6(8): e04433.
[http://dx.doi.org/10.1016/j.heliyon.2020.e04433] [PMID: 32775740]

[22] Yi PH, Wei J, Kim TK, *et al.* Automated detection & classification of knee arthroplasty using deep learning. Knee 2020; 27(2): 535-42.
[http://dx.doi.org/10.1016/j.knee.2019.11.020] [PMID: 31883760]

[23] Knipe H, Pai V. Kellgren and Lawrence system for classification of osteoarthritis. 2014. Available from: https://radiopaedia.org/articles/kellgren-and-lawrence-system-for-classification-of-osteoarthritis (updated 2021 Sep 15; cited 2022 Sep 26).

[24] Audrey HX, Abd Razak HRB, Andrew THC. The truth behind subchondral cysts in osteoarthritis of the knee. Open Orthop J 2014; 8(1): 7-10.
[http://dx.doi.org/10.2174/1874325001408010007] [PMID: 24533038]

[25] Kohn MD, Sassoon AA, Fernando ND. Classifications in brief: Kellgren-lawrence classification of osteoarthritis. Clin Orthop Relat Res 2016; 474(8): 1886-93.
[http://dx.doi.org/10.1007/s11999-016-4732-4] [PMID: 26872913]

[26] Gonçalves FB, Rocha FA, Albuquerque RP, Mozella AP, Crespo B, Cobra H. Reproducibility assessment of different descriptions of the Kellgren and Lawrence classification for osteoarthritis of the knee. Revista Brasileira de Ortopedia 2016; 51(6): 687-91.
[http://dx.doi.org/10.1016/j.rboe.2016.10.009] [PMID: 28050541]

[27] Stern AG, Moxley G, Sudha Rao TP, *et al.* Utility of digital photographs of the hand for assessing the presence of hand osteoarthritis. Osteoarthritis Cartilage 2004; 12(5): 360-5.
[http://dx.doi.org/10.1016/j.joca.2004.01.003] [PMID: 15094134]

[28] Vos T, Flaxman AD, Naghavi M, *et al.* Years lived with disability (YLDs) for 1160 sequelae of 289 diseases and injuries 1990–2010: A systematic analysis for the Global Burden of Disease Study 2010. Lancet 2012; 380(9859): 2163-96.
[http://dx.doi.org/10.1016/S0140-6736(12)61729-2] [PMID: 23245607]

[29] Osteoarthritis Initiative. National Institute of Arthritis and Musculoskeletal and Skin Diseases. 2004. Available from: https://www.niams.nih.gov/grants-funding/funded-research/osteoarthritis-initiative (updated 2020 July; cited 2022 Sep 26).

[30] Multicenter Osteoarthritis Study (MOST). National Institute on Aging. Available from: https://www.nia.nih.gov/research/resource/multicenter-osteoarthritis-study-most (cited 2022 Sep 26).

CHAPTER 3

Role of Cytokines and Chemokines in Rheumatoid Arthritis

Hanan Hassan Omar[1,*]

[1] *Clinical Pathology Department, Faculty of Medicine, Suez Canal University, Ismailia, Egypt*

Abstract: Rheumatoid arthritis (RA) is a chronic, inflammatory, and destructive polyarthritis with numerous autoimmune features and the potential for extra-articular and systemic complications. Much progress has occurred in defining important mechanistic components of RA, leading to significant advances in its treatment. RA is a multifactorial and multistage disease, beginning with preclinical autoimmunity that arises in a genetically predisposed individual who encounters one or more environmental triggers, progressing to the clinical appearance of inflammation in joints and sometimes in other organs, and leading to destruction of the articular cartilage and adjacent bone. Regulatory role in inflammation, autoimmunity and articular destruction in the joints of rheumatoid arthritis patients is played primarily by chemokines and cytokines. Amongst many top players of inflammation in RA, tumour-necrosis factor-alpha (TNF-α) is counted as the chief culprit. It is produced by synovial macrophages, B lymphocytes, and NK-cells. Furthermore, TNF-α has exhibited to be of particular utility as a therapeutic target. IL-17A is synthesized by T helper 17 (Th17), which initiates the generation of inflammation causing cytokines like interleukin-6 (IL-6), IL-8 and GM-CSF by cells of endothelium, epithelium and fibroblasts and localization of neutrophils. Progression of inflammation in the synovial fluid is augmented by chemokines in the joints of rheumatoid patients. Elevated levels of CC chemokines (CCL2, CCL3, CCL4 and CCL5) and CXC chemokines (CXCL5, CXCL8, CXCL9 and CXCL10) have been reported in such patients. Moreover, these chemokines may control cell trafficking directly by interacting with their cognate receptors present on inflammatory cells and also by modulating angiogenesis. Several proinflammatory cytokines and chemokines participate in many biological pathways finally setting the loop of inflammation and exacerbation of the outcome and these serve as biomarkers for a number of autoimmune and inflammatory disorders.

Keywords: Rheumatoid arthritis, Cytokines, Chemokine.

* **Corresponding author Hanan Hassan Omar:** Clinical Pathology Department, Faculty of Medicine, Suez Canal University, Ismailia, Egypt; Tel: +20-1093627403; E-mail: hananhassan1978@gmail.com

Puneetpal Singh (Ed.)

INTRODUCTION

Rheumatoid arthritis (RA) is a chronic autoimmune disease characterized by a communication between innate and adaptive immune cells and mediators. Such cellular cross talks are responsible for triggering systemic as well as local at different phases of this disease. It has been documented that almost 0.2-1 percent of North Americans and Europeans are suffering from RA, however, considerable regional variation is noticed. Moreover, incidence rates for RA were observed to be approximately 500 patients per 100,000 populations with considerable geographical incongruity [1].

In recent years, researchers have made significant progress in understanding the mechanisms involving cells from both the innate and adaptive immune systems, such as monocytes and macrophages [2, 3]. By orchestrating various inflammatory and tissue remodeling pathways, many soluble and membrane-bound mediators play important roles in this cross-talk [4, 5].

Inflammatory cytokines are capable of activating destructive mechanisms in the joint, resulting in structural damage and, as a result, a functional reduction in mobility which ends with disability [6]. The complicated interactions of inflammatory cytokines are responsible for joint injury that begins at the synovial membrane and proceeds to other joint tissues [7]. There is widespread activation of monocytes, macrophages, and synovial fibroblasts, as well as an increase in the production of proinflammatory cytokines such as Interleukin 1(IL-1), Interleukin 6(IL-6), and Tumor-necrosis factor-alpha (TNF-α) [8]. Other cytokines and chemokines that are detected in the synovial membrane include Interleukin 15 (IL-15), Interleukin 17 (IL-17), and Interleukin 18 (IL-18). These inflammatory cytokines activate various signaling pathways and stimulate gene transcription, which are important factors in inflammation and the degradation of the tissue [9].

The inflammation causing cytokines are the key targets to control RA. TNF-targeting has been shown to be effective in the treatment of RA using either customized cytokine antibodies or used as receptors for soluble cytokines as decoys. Pro-inflammatory cytokine activity can even be inhibited by small molecule inhibitors of cytokine signaling or by utilizing targeted short interfering RNA (siRNA) to suppress the expression of a specific cytokine [10].

B cells in the peripheral blood of RA patients can secrete many cytokines including Chemokine (C-C motif) ligand 3(CCL3), TNF-α, Interferon gamma (IFN-γ), IL-6, Interleukin-1β (IL-1β), IL-17, and IL-18. TNF-α can increase the expression of receptor activator of nuclear factor-κB ligand (RANKL) by B cells in the presence of IL-1β, thereby promoting the formation of osteoclasts [11, 12] (Fig. **1**). Regulatory B (Breg) cells are a type of B cells that exert immunosuppressive functions. Breg cells are mainly responsible for the production of anti-inflammatory cytokines (IL-10, TGF-β, and IL-35) [13].

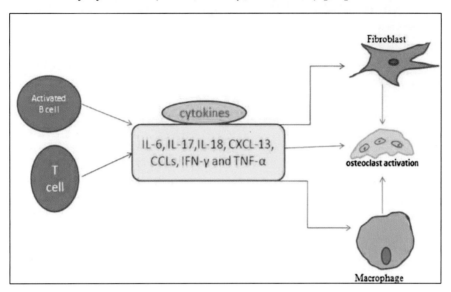

Fig. (1). Cytokine secretion by B cells in RA.

ROLE AND RELEVANCE OF CYTOKINES IN RA PATHOGENESIS

Cytokines play a pivotal role in the development of RA inflammation due to their role as signaling molecules between immune cells and tissue cells. TNF-α, IL-17A, IFN-γ and receptor activator of nuclear factor κB ligand are the most common but prominent cytokines formed by invading T cells (RANK-L) [14].

Amongst many top most promising mediators of joint inflammation in RA, TNF-α is counted as chief culprit. It is produced by synovial macrophages, B-cells, and Natural killer (NK) cells. TNF-α is found largely in biopsy specimens of arthritic tissue and its exaggeration causes natural inflammation in a variety of mouse models of arthritis. It may cause severe degradation of cartilage and bone, according to early *in vitro* investigations [15].

TNF-α has been found to induce osteoclast genesis by increasing RANK-L production by osteocytes. According to some studies, it may also directly drive the development of monocyte/macrophage lineage cells into osteoclasts *via* a RANK-L-independent mechanism [12, 16]. The potential of TNF-α to increase the production of other inflammatory cytokines, such as IL-1β and IL-6, which invite leukocytes and encourage the creation of an inflammatory environment in the synovial fluid, is another key role of TNF-α in the pathogenesis of RA [17].

T helper 17 cells (Th17 cells) generate IL-17A, which stimulates the production of pro-inflammatory cytokines such as IL-6, IL-8, and granulocyte-macrophage colony-stimulating factor (GM-CSF) by epithelial, endothelial, and fibroblastic cells, as well as neutrophil recruitment, resulting in local inflammation and disease development. IL-17A plays a role in bone attrition, cartilage deterioration and angiogenesis in RA pathogenesis. IL-17A causes osteoclast progenitors to grow into mature osteoclasts and stimulates the synthesis of RANK-L by the involvement of bone cells; osteoblasts and synoviocytes finally leading to decreased bone acrual and increased bone degradation [18].

Furthermore, IL-17A has been demonstrated to encourage synoviocytes to increase the production of matrix metalloproteinase (MMP)-1 ultimately causing cartilage degradation. In the pathophysiology of RA, angiogenesis is crucial. IL-17A has been found to promote endothelial cell migration as well as the generation of vascular endothelial growth factor (VEGF) by employing synovial fibroblasts [19].

IFN-γ is another significant cytokine in the pathogenesis of RA. It is found in large amounts in the plasma, synovial tissue, and synovial fluid of RA patients. T cells, B cells, NK cells, monocytes/macrophages, Dendritic cells (DCs), and neutrophil granulocytes all produce IFN-γ [20]. It binds to the ubiquitously expressed IFN-γ receptor, triggering the activation of IFN-γ stimulated genes through a variety of pathways, including the Janus activated kinase–signal transducer and activator of transcription 1 (JAK–STAT1) pathway, as well as the mitogen activated protein (MAP) kinase–, phosphatidylinositol 3-kinase (PI3K), and nuclear factor κb [21].

IFN- γ stimulated monocytes and macrophages which release C-X-C motif chemokine ligand 10 (CXCL10), a chemokine that promotes osteoclast development by stimulating RANK-L and TNF-α production from CD4+ T cells. As a result, IFN-γ contributes to the formation of early inflammation in RA [22]. In addition, IFN-γ has an important role in the protection of tissue specifically in advanced stages of the disease through down-regulation and inhibition of the RANK–RANK-L-mediated osteoclastogenesis and many immunological processes such as neutrophil influx, TNFα-dependent synoviocytes proliferation, production of degrading enzymes, synthesis of prostaglandin E2 as well as granulocyte-macrophage colony-stimulating factor (GM-CSF) [21].

Cytokines are cell-produced proteins that act as molecular messengers across cells. In arthritis, cytokines control numerous inflammatory responses. The classification of cytokines is essential to know the structure and function of each cytokine. The cytokines are divided into many categories and classes including mainly chemokines, lymphokines and interleukins (ILs) and also tumor necrosis factors (TNFs), interferons (IFNs), monokines, colony stimulating factors (CSFs), and transforming growth factors (TGFs) were added. There are two types of inflammatory cytokines: ones that cause acute inflammation, such as IL-1, TNF-α, IL-6, IL-11, IL-8, and other chemokines, playing important roles in mediating acute inflammatory reactions. The other type are those that cause chronic inflammation which are further divided into the cytokines causing humeral inflammation as IL-3, IL-4, IL-5, IL-6, IL-7, IL-9, IL-10, IL-13, and transforming growth factor-beta (TGF-β), and the cytokines contributing to cellular inflammation as IL-1, IL-2, IL-3, IL-4, IL-7, IL-9, IL-10, IL-12, interferons (IFNs), IFN-γ inducing factor (IGIF), TGF-β, and TNF-α and -β. Based on the role of cytokines, these can be classified as pro-inflammatory or anti-inflammatory [23]. Pro-inflammatory cytokines, such as IL-1β, IL-6, IL-8, IL-12, TNF-α, and interferons, promote inflammatory responses and boost immunocompetent cells. Anti-inflammatory cytokines such as IL-4, IL-6, IL-10, IL-11, IL-13, IL-1 receptor antagonist (IL-1RA) and TGF, on the other hand mitigate inflammation and subdue immune system. IL-6 plays the role of both pro-inflammation and anti-inflammation [24].

Cytokines are the first to respond in inflammation and generate phase response for the protection of host against infection and injury. The synthesis of cytokines (IL-1, IL-6, IL-8, IL12, IFN-γ and TNF-α) from the identical or distinct cells initiates this reaction. The primary function of the produced cytokines is that these convey the presence of infection or injury to surrounding tissues. Furthermore, the effects of cytokines on the host circulation lead to many major changes through activating the host immune cells which represented as fever and the acute-phase reaction [24].

Another principle immunological function of pro-inflammatory cytokines is the protection of the host from the external infection with bacteria and any microorganisms as well as the endogenous flora of the skin and digestive system. Interestingly, macrophages are the main sources of pro-inflammatory cytokines which have a great and essential role in infection defense by initiating the activation of the adaptive immunity [25].

Unfortunately, chronic inflammation could occur resulting from the increased production of pro-inflammatory cytokines which result in many dangerous conditions and chronic illnesses, such as diabetes, cardiovascular diseases, gastrointestinal diseases, cancer and aging-related diseases [26, 27]. Numerous great publications have studied the critical roles of inflammatory cytokines in many immune disorders such as autoimmune conditions [28 - 31]. Santamaria discusses the influences of inflammatory cytokines and chemokines on a variety of autoimmune disorders [32]. Interferons that promote inflammation are critical in the expansion of autoimmune disorders. Some reports have highlighted the involvement of IFN-γ in the etiology of autoimmune illness, as well as its effect on affiliated morbid conditions and therapeutic interventional effects in the diseases of malignancy [33, 34].

Furthermore, inflammation augmenting cytokines activate adhesion molecules and metalloproteinases, allowing for unique methods of tumour invasion. Such extreme inflammation causing reactions must be managed and regulated as a whole, or they may result in pathogenic conditions associated with the abnormal production of immune mediators [35].

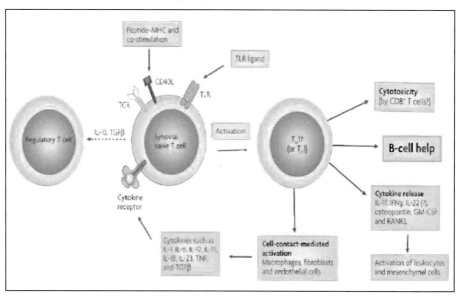

Fig. (2). The effector pathways of T cell activation in RA.

Synovial T cells may directly contribute to synovitis by producing inflammatory cytokines (Fig. **2**). T-cell-derived IL-17 has an effector role. IL-17 promotes neutrophil differentiation, maturation, activation, and cytokine release, as well as monocyte activation, synovial fibroblast activation, chemokine release, prostaglandin generation, and MMP synthesis. It is also possible that IL-17 and TNF-γ will activate DCs in the joint. A synergistic impact with modest amounts of IL-17, IL-1, and TNF-γ has also been demonstrated, which results in synovial fibroblast activation and cytokine production, indicating a pathogenic function for these inflammatory cascades. It is increasingly becoming obvious that Th17 cells may exert their effects *via* other cytokines [36]. IL-22, (IL-10-family member), is generated by activation of Th17 cells *via* IL-6 or IL-23 cytokines to increase skin inflammation and modify cutaneous acanthosis. In the synovial membranes of rheumatoid arthritis patients, IL-22 and its receptor were established, however, IL-22 was linked with CD68+cells as an alternate of T cells, revealing macrophages or synovial fibroblasts [37].

This could be due to TGF-β inhibiting Th17 cell synthesis of IL-22. TGF-β has equivocal inflammatory effects in synovitis: in the presence of IL-6, it can stimulate cell differentiation into Th17 cells, however, in IL-6 deficiency, the generation of T cells with a regulatory phenotype was enhanced. The inflammatory cytokines derive from T-cell, as Osteopontin, could also have a pivotal role. The cytokine, osteopontin, can bind to multiple integrins including CD44 [38].

Interestingly, Osteopontin expression has been found in the synovial membrane of RA patients. In the RA joints, synovial CD4+ T cells appear to operate as a paracrine and autocrine amplification factor for cytokine release, stimulating the synthesis of IL-1 and other chemokines. Additionally, synovial inflammation could be occurred through the direct activation of fibroblasts and macrophages *via* nearby T- cells interaction. Also, TNF and IL-1β production from syngeneic macrophages is thus induced by freshly isolated synovial T cells in a cell-contact-dependent manner [39].

With regard to effector profile and the signal cascade that they create inside macrophages, such cytokine-activated T cells closely mirror those identified in the synovium, indicating that this may be an essential mechanism for sustaining cytokine release *in vivo*. Importantly, the T cell's activation status (that is, T cell receptor (TCR) ligation or cytokine activation) and phenotype (Th1 or Th2) determine which signaling pathways (such as PI3K versus nuclear factor-B (NF-B) activation) are triggered in target macrophages, and which cytokines and chemokines are released by target macrophages [35, 40]. The receptor-ligand combinations identified in T-cell–macrophage interactions are unclear, but they include CD40–CD40L (CD40 ligand), LFA1–ICAM1 (lymphocyte function-associated antigen 1–intercellular adhesion molecule 1), CD2–LFA3 and CD69. In paracrine regulatory loops, IL-4, IL-10, and TGF, as well as apolipoprotein A1, can decrease T-cell–macrophage interactions. Synovial fibroblasts are triggered by reciprocal associations with activated T cells, mostly *via* T-cell transmission of membrane-bound cytokines to synovial fibroblasts, suggesting that this is a general effector mechanism in chronic inflammation [41].

ROLE OF ANTI-INFLAMMATORY CYTOKINES

There are many established anti-inflammatory cytokines. They have an important role in immunological inflammatory response. The immune-regulatory molecules as IL-1 receptor antagonists, IL-4, IL-6, IL-10, IL-11, IL-13, and TGF-β reduce the excessive inflammatory response resulting from inflammation causing cytokines. IL-10, a powerful inflammation protecting cytokine, has immune-regulatory effects which can prevent the effect of various reported pro-inflammatory cytokines through decreasing its releasing amounts from the immune cells. There are anti-inflammatory effects of IL-10 on many immune cells such as Basophils, eosinophils and mast cells. It has an important role in the management and regulation of allergies and asthma. Anti-inflammatory cytokines have been found to have physiological characteristics [30].

Cytokines prevent the potentially harmful effects of prolonged or excessive inflammatory triggering responses. Inflammation controlling cytokines have been useful in many diseases linked with augmented inflammation. These can be employed as medicines to resolve inflammation-related disorders. However, in comparison to anti-inflammatory medications such as neutralizing antidotes, cytokine treatment has a number of drawbacks [31]. Some particular anti-inflammatory mediators may successfully reduce arthritic burden by influencing innate immunity cells or by meddling with B and T cell activation. Inflammation protection cytokine; IL-35 regulates the role of T cell and attenuates pathogenic cells like Th1 and Th17 cells, hence reducing the brutality of collagen-triggered arthritis [42]. However, the immune response is stalled resulting in the vulnerability of host towards systemic infection. Although research shows that endogenous IL-10 protects against severe sepsis by lowering TNF synthesis, excessive IL-10 production leading to increased TNF inhibition may be harmful due to the decrease of TNF's antibacterial action [32].

Finally, multiple cytokines are associated with various biological states, and they serve as biological markers for a number of inflammatory and auto-immune disorders [33].

ROLE AND RELEVANCE OF CHEMOKINES IN RA PATHOGENESIS

Many chemokines perform important roles in development, homeostasis, and function of the immune system. Sidewise from chemotaxis, chemokines are known to have further functions, including roles in cell proliferation, angiogenesis, and T-cell differentiation. Chemokines are also key players in inflammation, and their levels could be significantly elevated in tissues and plasma of patients with inflammatory conditions. Additionally, there are well established associations between chemokines and different diseases such as rheumatoid arthritis, asthma, and psoriasis [43].

In arthritis, leukocytes extravasate through the vascular endothelium into the synovial tissue. Numerous synovial chemotactic mediators termed chemokines and their receptors are involved in this process. There are more than 50 known chemokines and 19 chemokine receptors. Some of these chemokines and chemokine receptors are also involved in intense synovial angiogenesis, the formation of new capillaries from preexisting vessels [44]. In RA, pro-inflammatory chemokines overrule anti-inflammatory chemokines resulting in accelerated inflammation in the synovial tissue. Elevated levels of CC chemokines (CCL2, CCL3, CCL4 and CCL5) and CXC chemokines (CXCL5, CXCL8, CXCL9 and CXCL10) have been reported for biological samples from RA patients [45]. Interestingly, these chemokines may control cell trafficking directly by interacting with their cognate receptors present on inflammatory cells and also by modulating angiogenesis [46]. CXC chemokines containing an ELR amino acid motif, such as CXCL5 and CXCL8, promote neovascularization, which allows sustained cell migration and the supply of oxygen and nutrients for the developing invasive 'pannus' (*i.e.* the inflammatory synovial tissue). The angiostatic chemokines CXCL9 and CXCL10 are also abundantly present in RA joints and may counteract the effects of the pro-angiogenic mediators [47].

Peripheral blood monocytes can be expressed in different types of CC and CXC receptors that can bind most of the pro-inflammatory chemokines. In RA patients, circulating monocytes have been found to express mainly CCR1, CCR2, and CCR4, whereas synovial fluid is enriched in CCR3+ and CCR5+ cells. Different laboratories have reported that CD4+ memory T cells from synovium express CCR5, CXCR2, CXCR3, CXCR4 and/or CXCR6 at higher levels than expressed by circulating T cells [47].

It has been observed that CXCL10 is present in serum, synovial tissue (ST) as well as synovial fluid (SF) in patients having RA and its levels are higher than in osteoarthritis patients. In addition, in synovial membrane of RA patients, it is primarily secreted by infiltrating macrophage like cells [48].

CXCL9 is frequently found in RA SF and ST, and mediates many inflammatory processes occurring in the synovium. Additionally, CXCL9 and CXCL10 are both CXC motif chemokine receptor-3 (CXCR3) binding ligands. These chemokines were released in response to IFN-γ stimulation. The expression of CXCR3 was commonly found in inflamed ST activated T-cell rich areas [49]. Moreover, it was associated with a high IFN γ/interleukin-4 ratio, suggesting Th1 activated rather than a Th2 phenotype [50].

CXCL10 may increase the expression of RANKL in RA synoviocytes and significantly heightened expression of RANKL in CD4+ T cells. It has been found that CXCL10 induces TRAP (tartrate-resistant acid phosphatase)-positive osteoclast differentiation in a dose-dependent manner. Moreover, osteoprotegerin (OPG) (a soluble RANKL antagonist) can inhibit this differentiation and also it could be suppressed *via* neutralizing anti-CXCL10 antibody. The effective anti-rheumatic biological treatment in RA is anti-TNF antibody and during using this treatment, the osteoclastogenesis was inhibited which induced by CXCL10. Consequently, these finding confirm the role of CXCL10 in stimulating osteoclast differentiation *via* RANKL and TNF-α expression [51].

Generally, in osteoclast precursors, RANKL promotes CXCL10 expression and *via* Gαi subunit of CXCR3. RANKL expression is regulated by the CXCL10 in CD4+ T cells in synovial cavity of RA patients [52]. Notably, the interaction of CXCL10 with RANKL, as well as with many inflammatory cytokines, could be the main reason of bone degradation and the initiation and/or worsening of inflammation RA (Fig. **3**).

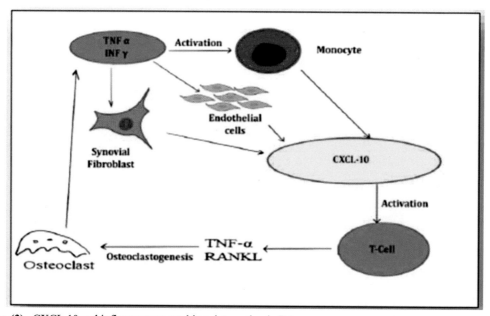

Fig. (3). CXCL-10 and inflammatory cytokines interaction in RA.

Earlier CXCR3 ligands were known as IFN-γ inducible genes which were present largely in either monocytes or macrophage lineage cells [53]. CXCR3 and their associated chemokines probably regulate the recruitment of macrophages and monocytes which play a role in inflammation. T cells present in synovium are observed to be strongly stained for CXCR3 in some immunofluorescence studies. Approximately 90% of CD4+ T cells which were observed to be present in the synovial fluid exhibit this receptor. T cells along with CXCR3 expressing mast cells and plasma cells exist in the infiltrated synovial soft tissue of RA patients [54].

Synovial fluid and soft tissue have been shown to harbor CXCR3-binding chemokines in extremely large quantities in RA patients. It has been documented by some studies that the synovial fibroblasts are the key players to produce three CXCR3 agonistic chemokines *i.e.* CXCL9, CXCL10, and CXCL11 when IFN-γ and TNF-α interact and play synergistically [55].

Beyond doubt, in RA, CXCR3 pathway is the chief culprit for joint inflammation. Studies have highlighted that therapeutic molecules like lipo-oxygenase dual inhibitors and cyclooxygenase prevent the synthesis of CXCR3 ligands by blocking synovial fibroblasts and TNF-α and change the course of trafficking of CXCR3+ T cells. It has been evident that synovial tissue of RA patients produces chemokines; CXCL9, CXCL10, CXCL11 in large quantities. Moreover, fibroblast cell lines within synovium of RA patients generate significant quantities of these chemokine proteins when poked by IFN-γ, Th1 cytokine along with inflammation triggering cytokine TNF-α [54].

Similarly higher levels of these chemokines are generated when a joint encounters inflammation. Furthermore, higher levels of CXCR3 agonists within plasma and synovium of RA patients reveal that these play collaboratively for the recruitment of T cells, especially Th1-type cells. In the synovial fluid of patients with RA, T-cells expressed high level of CXCR3 and CXCl10 detected by immune-staining. The levels of these chemokines were more elevated in the synovium then the levels in blood [53].

CXCL13, (C-X-C motif chemokine ligand 13), known as B lymphocyte chemoattractant (BLC) or B cell-attracting chemokine 1 (BCA-1), is expressed by follicular dendritic cells and macrophages acting through its known receptor CXCR5 (C-X-C motif chemokine 5), on mature B cells and a subset of T helper cells. The over-activation of CXCL13/CXCR5 signaling axis has been reported to be involved in inflammatory, infectious, lympho-proliferative disorders as well as immune responses. It has been proven to have an important role in the pathogenesis of many autoimmune diseases including rheumatoid arthritis, autoimmune thyroiditis, SLE, and others [56].

In RA, the Serum CXCL13 levels were highly increased. The degree of elevation was associated with elevated in rheumatoid factor (RF) positive and anti-citrullinated peptide antibodies (ACPA) positive. In addition, CXCL13 was strongly associated with both IgM and IgA RA [57].

Moreover, increased levels of CXCL13 were associated with joint damage and RA disease activity. Consequently, CXCL13 levels were correlated with the markers of activity such as tender joints, erythrocyte sedimentation rate (ESR) and C-reactive protein (CRP) [14].

CXCL13 was expressed in synovial fluids (SF) in RA patients. Additionally, this expression was associated with bone degradation resulting from immune cell activation. Consequently, CXCL13 could be used as a predictor of the severity of the RA disease and also can diagnose erosive RA [43].

CONCLUSION

Rheumatoid arthritis disease is a common autoimmune inflammatory disease which affects small joints. Many cytokines and chemokines have crucial roles in RA pathogenesis and activate damaging mechanisms in the joint, resulting in structural damage and, functional reduction in mobility and end with disability. Interestingly, these cytokines and chemokines are associated with various biological states, and they serve as diagnostic biomarkers and could be particularly used as therapeutic targets in RA disease.

REFERENCES

[1]   Almutairi K, Nossent J, Preen D, Keen H, Inderjeeth C. The global prevalence of rheumatoid arthritis: A meta-analysis based on a systematic review. Rheumatol Int 2021; 41(5): 863-77.
[http://dx.doi.org/10.1007/s00296-020-04731-0] [PMID: 33175207]

[2]   Acevedo OA, Berrios RV, Rodríguez-Guilarte L, Lillo-Dapremont B, Kalergis AM. molecular and cellular mechanisms modulating trained immunity by various cell types in response to pathogen encounter. Front Immunol 2021; 12: 745332.
[http://dx.doi.org/10.3389/fimmu.2021.745332] [PMID: 34671359]

[3]   Austermann J, Roth J, Barczyk-Kahlert K. The good and the bad: Monocytes' and macrophages' diverse functions in inflammation. Cells 2022; 11(12): 1979.
[http://dx.doi.org/10.3390/cells11121979] [PMID: 35741108]

[4]   Giannini D, Antonucci M, Petrelli F, Bilia S, Alunno A, Puxeddu I. One year in review 2020: Pathogenesis of rheumatoid arthritis. Clin Exp Rheumatol 2020; 38(3): 387-97.
[http://dx.doi.org/10.55563/clinexprheumatol/3uj1ng] [PMID: 32324123]

[5]   Testa D, Calvacchi S, Petrelli F, *et al.* One year in review 2021: Pathogenesis of rheumatoid arthritis. Clin Exp Rheumatol 2021; 39(3): 445-52.
[http://dx.doi.org/10.55563/clinexprheumatol/j115l3] [PMID: 34018918]

[6]   Chen L, Deng H, Cui H, *et al.* Inflammatory responses and inflammation-associated diseases in organs. Oncotarget 2018; 9(6): 7204-18.
[http://dx.doi.org/10.18632/oncotarget.23208] [PMID: 29467962]

[7]   Dwivedi G, Flaman L, Alaybeyoglu B, *et al.* Inflammatory cytokines and mechanical injury induce post-traumatic osteoarthritis-like changes in a human cartilage-bone-synovium microphysiological system. Arthritis Res Ther 2022; 24(1): 198.
[http://dx.doi.org/10.1186/s13075-022-02881-z] [PMID: 35982461]

[8]   McInnes IB, Schett G. Cytokines in the pathogenesis of rheumatoid arthritis. Nat Rev Immunol 2007; 7(6): 429-42.
[http://dx.doi.org/10.1038/nri2094] [PMID: 17525752]

[9]   Firestein GS. Evolving concepts of rheumatoid arthritis. Nature 2003; 423(6937): 356-61.
[http://dx.doi.org/10.1038/nature01661] [PMID: 12748655]

[10]   Venkatesha S, Dudics S, Acharya B, Moudgil K. Cytokine-modulating strategies and newer cytokine targets for arthritis therapy. Int J Mol Sci 2014; 16(1): 887-906.

[http://dx.doi.org/10.3390/ijms16010887] [PMID: 25561237]

[11]   Zhao B. Intrinsic restriction of TNF-mediated inflammatory osteoclastogenesis and bone resorption. Front Endocrinol 2020; 11: 583561.
[http://dx.doi.org/10.3389/fendo.2020.583561] [PMID: 33133025]

[12]   Jura-Półtorak A, Szeremeta A, Olczyk K, Zoń-Giebel A, Komosińska-Vassev K. Bone metabolism and RANKL/OPG ratio in rheumatoid arthritis women treated with TNF-α inhibitors. J Clin Med 2021; 10(13): 2905.
[http://dx.doi.org/10.3390/jcm10132905] [PMID: 34209821]

[13]   Wu H, Chen S, Li A, *et al.* LncRNA expression profiles in systemic lupus erythematosus and rheumatoid arthritis: Emerging biomarkers and therapeutic targets. Front Immunol 2021; 12: 792884.
[http://dx.doi.org/10.3389/fimmu.2021.792884] [PMID: 35003113]

[14]   Smolen JS, Aletaha D, Barton A, *et al.* Rheumatoid arthritis. Nat Rev Dis Primers 2018; 4(1): 18001.
[http://dx.doi.org/10.1038/nrdp.2018.1] [PMID: 29417936]

[15]   Ma H, Xu M, Song Y, Zhang T, Yin H, Yin S. Interferon-γ facilitated adjuvant-induced arthritis at early stage. Scand J Immunol 2019; 89(5): e12757.
[http://dx.doi.org/10.1111/sji.12757] [PMID: 30739356]

[16]   Hu Y, Li X, Zhi X, *et al.* RANKL from bone marrow adipose lineage cells promotes osteoclast formation and bone loss. EMBO Rep 2021; 22(7): e52481.
[http://dx.doi.org/10.15252/embr.202152481] [PMID: 34121311]

[17]   Marahleh A, Kitaura H, Ohori F, *et al.* TNF-α directly enhances osteocyte RANKL expression and promotes osteoclast formation. Front Immunol 2019; 10: 2925.
[http://dx.doi.org/10.3389/fimmu.2019.02925] [PMID: 31921183]

[18]   Robert M, Miossec P. IL-17 in rheumatoid arthritis and precision medicine: From synovitis expression to circulating bioactive levels. Front Med 2019; 5: 364.
[http://dx.doi.org/10.3389/fmed.2018.00364] [PMID: 30693283]

[19]   Lin YJ, Anzaghe M, Schülke S. Update on the pathomechanism, diagnosis, and treatment options for rheumatoid arthritis. Cells 2020; 9(4): 880.
[http://dx.doi.org/10.3390/cells9040880] [PMID: 32260219]

[20]   Thanapati S, Ganu M, Giri P, *et al.* Impaired NK cell functionality and increased TNF-α production as biomarkers of chronic chikungunya arthritis and rheumatoid arthritis. Hum Immunol 2017; 78(4): 370-4.
[http://dx.doi.org/10.1016/j.humimm.2017.02.006] [PMID: 28213049]

[21]   Tang M, Tian L, Luo G, Yu X. Interferon-gamma-mediated osteoimmunology. Front Immunol 2018; 9: 1508.
[http://dx.doi.org/10.3389/fimmu.2018.01508] [PMID: 30008722]

[22]   Olalekan SA, Cao Y, Hamel KM, Finnegan A. B cells expressing IFN-γ suppress Treg-cell differentiation and promote autoimmune experimental arthritis. Eur J Immunol 2015; 45(4): 988-98.
[http://dx.doi.org/10.1002/eji.201445036] [PMID: 25645456]

[23]   Sprague AH, Khalil RA. Inflammatory cytokines in vascular dysfunction and vascular disease. Biochem Pharmacol 2009; 78(6): 539-52.
[http://dx.doi.org/10.1016/j.bcp.2009.04.029] [PMID: 19413999]

[24]   Boshtam M, Asgary S, Kouhpayeh S, Shariati L, Khanahmad H. Aptamers against pro- and anti-inflammatory cytokines: A Review. Inflammation 2017; 40(1): 340-9.
[http://dx.doi.org/10.1007/s10753-016-0477-1] [PMID: 27878687]

[25]   Cheng A, Yan H, Han C, Wang W, Tian Y, Chen X. Polyphenols from blueberries modulate inflammation cytokines in LPS-induced RAW264.7 macrophages. Int J Biol Macromol 2014; 69: 382-7.
[http://dx.doi.org/10.1016/j.ijbiomac.2014.05.071] [PMID: 24905959]

[26]   Mendes V, Galvão I, Vieira AT. Mechanisms by which the gut microbiota influences cytokine production and modulates host inflammatory responses. J Interferon Cytokine Res 2019; 39(7): 393-409.
[http://dx.doi.org/10.1089/jir.2019.0011] [PMID: 31013453]

[27]   Lin CH, Chen CC, Chiang HL, *et al.* Altered gut microbiota and inflammatory cytokine responses in patients with Parkinson's disease. J Neuroinflammation 2019; 16(1): 129.
[http://dx.doi.org/10.1186/s12974-019-1528-y] [PMID: 31248424]

[28]   Kany S, Vollrath JT, Relja B. Cytokines in inflammatory disease. Int J Mol Sci 2019; 20(23): 6008.
[http://dx.doi.org/10.3390/ijms20236008] [PMID: 31795299]

[29]   Niu X, Chen G. Clinical biomarkers and pathogenic-related cytokines in rheumatoid arthritis. J Immunol Res 2014; 2014: 1-7.
[http://dx.doi.org/10.1155/2014/698192] [PMID: 25215307]

[30]   Rodney T, Osier N, Gill J. Pro- and anti-inflammatory biomarkers and traumatic brain injury outcomes: A review. Cytokine 2018; 110: 248-56.
[http://dx.doi.org/10.1016/j.cyto.2018.01.012] [PMID: 29396048]

[31]   Raphael I, Nalawade S, Eagar TN, Forsthuber TG. T cell subsets and their signature cytokines in autoimmune and inflammatory diseases. Cytokine 2015; 74(1): 5-17.
[http://dx.doi.org/10.1016/j.cyto.2014.09.011] [PMID: 25458968]

[32]   Santamaria P. Cytokines and chemokines in autoimmune disease: an overview. Adv Exp Med Biol 2003; 520: 1-7.
[http://dx.doi.org/10.1007/978-1-4615-0171-8_1] [PMID: 12613569]

[33]   Hodge DL, Berthet C, Coppola V, *et al.* IFN-gamma AU-rich element removal promotes chronic IFN-gamma expression and autoimmunity in mice. J Autoimmun 2014; 53: 33-45.
[http://dx.doi.org/10.1016/j.jaut.2014.02.003] [PMID: 24583068]

[34]   Bae HR, Leung PSC, Tsuneyama K, *et al.* Chronic expression of interferon-gamma leads to murine autoimmune cholangitis with a female predominance. Hepatology 2016; 64(4): 1189-201.
[http://dx.doi.org/10.1002/hep.28641] [PMID: 27178326]

[35]   Lawrence T. The nuclear factor NF-kappaB pathway in inflammation. Cold Spring Harb Perspect Biol 2009; 1(6): a001651.
[http://dx.doi.org/10.1101/cshperspect.a001651] [PMID: 20457564]

[36]   Steinman L. A brief history of TH17, the first major revision in the TH1/TH2 hypothesis of T cell–mediated tissue damage. Nat Med 2007; 13(2): 139-45.
[http://dx.doi.org/10.1038/nm1551] [PMID: 17290272]

[37]   Ikeuchi H, Kuroiwa T, Hiramatsu N, *et al.* Expression of interleukin-22 in rheumatoid arthritis: Potential role as a proinflammatory cytokine. Arthritis Rheum 2005; 52(4): 1037-46.
[http://dx.doi.org/10.1002/art.20965] [PMID: 15818686]

[38]   Yumoto K, Ishijima M, Rittling SR, *et al.* Osteopontin deficiency protects joints against destruction in anti-type II collagen antibody-induced arthritis in mice. Proc Natl Acad Sci 2002; 99(7): 4556-61.
[http://dx.doi.org/10.1073/pnas.052523599] [PMID: 11930008]

[39]   Xu G, Nie H, Li N, *et al.* Role of osteopontin in amplification and perpetuation of rheumatoid synovitis. J Clin Invest 2005; 115(4): 1060-7.
[http://dx.doi.org/10.1172/JCI200523273] [PMID: 15761492]

[40]   Shah K, Al-Haidari A, Sun J, Kazi JU. T cell receptor (TCR) signaling in health and disease. Signal Transduct Target Ther 2021; 6(1): 412.
[http://dx.doi.org/10.1038/s41392-021-00823-w] [PMID: 34897277]

[41]   Dayer JM, Burger D. Cell-cell interactions and tissue damage in rheumatoid arthritis. Autoimmun Rev 2004; 3 (1): S14-6.

[PMID: 15309769]

[42]   Ye C, Yano H, Workman CJ, Vignali DAA. Interleukin-35: Structure, function and its impact on immune-related diseases. J Interferon Cytokine Res 2021; 41(11): 391-406.
[http://dx.doi.org/10.1089/jir.2021.0147] [PMID: 34788131]

[43]   Mueller AL, Payandeh Z, Mohammadkhani N, *et al.* Recent advances in understanding the pathogenesis of rheumatoid arthritis: New treatment strategies. Cells 2021; 10(11): 3017.
[http://dx.doi.org/10.3390/cells10113017] [PMID: 34831240]

[44]   MacDonald I, Liu SC, Su CM, Wang YH, Tsai CH, Tang CH. Implications of angiogenesis involvement in arthritis. Int J Mol Sci 2018; 19(7): 2012.
[http://dx.doi.org/10.3390/ijms19072012] [PMID: 29996499]

[45]   Skrzypkowska M, Stasiak M, Sakowska J, *et al.* Cytokines and chemokines multiplex analysis in patients with low disease activity rheumatoid arthritis. Rheumatol Int 2022; 42(4): 609-19.
[http://dx.doi.org/10.1007/s00296-022-05103-6] [PMID: 35179632]

[46]   Szekanecz Z, Pakozdi A, Szentpetery A, Besenyei T, Koch AE. Chemokines and angiogenesis in rheumatoid arthritis. Front Biosci 2009; 1(1): 44-51.
[PMID: 19482623]

[47]   Szekanecz Z, Vegvari A, Szabo Z, Koch AE. Chemokines and chemokine receptors in arthritis. Front Biosci 2010; S2(1): 153-67.
[http://dx.doi.org/10.2741/s53] [PMID: 20036936]

[48]   Askenasy EM, Askenasy N. Is autoimmune diabetes caused by aberrant immune activity or defective suppression of physiological self-reactivity? Autoimmun Rev 2013; 12(5): 633-7.
[http://dx.doi.org/10.1016/j.autrev.2012.12.004] [PMID: 23277162]

[49]   Tozzoli R, Barzilai O, Ram M, *et al.* Infections and autoimmune thyroid diseases: Parallel detection of antibodies against pathogens with proteomic technology. Autoimmun Rev 2008; 8(2): 112-5.
[http://dx.doi.org/10.1016/j.autrev.2008.07.013] [PMID: 18700170]

[50]   Antonelli A, Ferrari SM, Giuggioli D, Ferrannini E, Ferri C, Fallahi P. Chemokine (C–X–C motif) ligand (CXCL)10 in autoimmune diseases. Autoimmun Rev 2014; 13(3): 272-80.
[http://dx.doi.org/10.1016/j.autrev.2013.10.010] [PMID: 24189283]

[51]   Lee E, Seo M, Juhnn YS, *et al.* Potential role and mechanism of IFN-gamma inducible protein-10 on receptor activator of nuclear factor kappa-B ligand (RANKL) expression in rheumatoid arthritis. Arthritis Res Ther 2011; 13(3): R104.
[http://dx.doi.org/10.1186/ar3385] [PMID: 21708014]

[52]   Lee JH, Kim B, Jin WJ, Kim HH, Ha H, Lee ZH. Pathogenic roles of CXCL10 signaling through CXCR3 and TLR4 in macrophages and T cells: relevance for arthritis. Arthritis Res Ther 2017; 19(1): 163.
[http://dx.doi.org/10.1186/s13075-017-1353-6] [PMID: 28724396]

[53]   Ueno A, Yamamura M, Iwahashi M, *et al.* The production of CXCR3-agonistic chemokines by synovial fibroblasts from patients with rheumatoid arthritis. Rheumatol Int 2005; 25(5): 361-7.
[http://dx.doi.org/10.1007/s00296-004-0449-x] [PMID: 15004722]

[54]   Lacotte S, Brun S, Muller S, Dumortier H. CXCR3, inflammation, and autoimmune diseases. Ann N Y Acad Sci 2009; 1173(1): 310-7.
[http://dx.doi.org/10.1111/j.1749-6632.2009.04813.x] [PMID: 19758167]

[55]   Tsubaki T, Takegawa S, Hanamoto H, *et al.* Accumulation of plasma cells expressing CXCR3 in the synovial sublining regions of early rheumatoid arthritis in association with production of Mig/CXCL9 by synovial fibroblasts. Clin Exp Immunol 2005; 141(2): 363-71.
[http://dx.doi.org/10.1111/j.1365-2249.2005.02850.x] [PMID: 15996201]

[56]   Kazanietz MG, Durando M, Cooke M. CXCL13 and Its Receptor CXCR5 in cancer: Inflammation, immune response, and beyond. Front Endocrinol 2019; 10: 471.

[http://dx.doi.org/10.3389/fendo.2019.00471] [PMID: 31354634]

[57]   Elemam NM, Hannawi S, Maghazachi AA. Role of chemokines and chemokine receptors in rheumatoid arthritis. ImmunoTargets Ther 2020; 9: 43-56.
[http://dx.doi.org/10.2147/ITT.S243636] [PMID: 32211348]

CHAPTER 4

Vitamin D and Immune System: Implications in Bone Health

Asha Bhardwaj[1], Tamanna Sharma[1], Sneha Das[1], Leena Sapra[1] and Rupesh K. Srivastava[1,*]

[1] Translational Immunology, Osteoimmunology & Immunoporosis Lab (TIOIL), Department of Biotechnology, All India Institute of Medical Sciences (AIIMS), New Delhi-110029, India

Abstract: Recent studies have identified the involvement of the immune system in several bone complications like osteoporosis, rheumatoid arthritis (RA), periodontitis, osteoarthritis, *etc.* Immune cells have an indispensable role in the regulation of bone metabolism and explicitly influence the differentiation of bone cells by producing various cytokines. Fortunately, recent research has examined different immune-based therapeutics for the prevention of bone diseases in addition to revealing more information about the interaction of the bone and the immune system. Vitamin D maintains bone health by effectively absorbing calcium and thereby promoting bone mineralization. In addition, vitamin D has great immunomodulatory potential and can influence the effect of immune cells and cytokines on the pathogenesis of bone deformities. Therefore, it is plausible to suggest that the detrimental effect of vitamin D deficiency on bone is also linked to the immune system apart from its classic effect on bone mineralization. However, very few studies have enlightened on this aspect of vitamin D-mediated regulation of bone homeostasis which needs to be further unraveled. In the present chapter, we have compiled recent studies highlighting the effect of vitamin D on bone health *via* its effect on the host immune system. Further, we have also highlighted the role of the immune system in the maintenance of skeletal health and then have discussed the effect of vitamin D on various immune cells. In addition, we have reviewed vitamin D-facilitated immune-based approaches for the effective management of various bone pathologies such as osteoporosis, osteoarthritis and rheumatoid arthritis. This information will supposedly help in revealing further mechanistic insights into the immunological regulation of bone health by vitamin D.

Keywords: Vitamin D, Osteoclasts, Osteoblasts, Osteocytes, Immune cells, Cytokines.

* **Corresponding author Rupesh K. Srivastava:** Translational Immunology, Osteoimmunology & Immunoporosis Lab (TIOIL), Department of Biotechnology, All India Institute of Medical Sciences (AIIMS), New Delhi-110029, India; Tel: +91-11-2659-3548; E-mail: rupesh_srivastava13@yahoo.co.in

Puneetpal Singh (Ed.)

INTRODUCTION

Bone is the metabolically active mineralized connective tissue that provides structural support, helps in muscle attachment for locomotion, safeguards the soft tissue, harbors bone marrow, and is the storehouse of calcium and phosphate [1]. Adult bone is composed of cortical and trabecular bone. Cortical bone is the solid dense compact bone surrounding the bone marrow. Cortical bone has a slow turnover rate and provides resistance to bending [2]. Trabecular bone on the other hand is flexible as it is less dense and has a high turnover rate. It consists of a honeycomb-like network of rods and plates that are interspersed in the bone marrow [2, 3]. Although the ratio of trabecular to cortical bone varies from bone to bone, an adult bone typically has 20% trabecular and 80% cortical bone [3]. Bone remodeling is the process through which bone is continuously modeled during the lifespan of an organism. Bone remodeling replaces the old bone with the new bone and is the result of coordinated action between the primary bone cells *i.e.* osteoclasts, osteoblasts, and osteocytes. Osteoclasts are bone-eating cells that are derived from the myeloid/monocyte hematopoietic lineage. During bone resorption, osteoclasts precursors are recruited towards the bone sites, where they fuse with each other to form the multinucleated osteoclasts that degrade calcified bone matrix by secreting various lytic and acidic enzymes [4]. Two necessary factors that are required for osteoclastogenesis are macrophage colony-stimulating factor (MCSF) and receptor activator of the nuclear factor kappa B ligand (RANKL). Both these factors are required for the expression of primary osteoclast markers such as cathepsin K, tartrate-resistant acid phosphatase (TRAP), calcitonin receptor, and beta 3 integrins. The binding of the RANKL to the RANK receptor on osteoclast precursors induces various changes such as rearrangement of the actin cytoskeleton and formation of tight junctions between the bone surface and basement membrane so that a sealed zone can be created. In this sealed zone (also known as resorption pit or Howship's lacunae), osteoclasts release various lytic enzymes such as TRAP and cathepsin K which lead to bone resorption. Enhanced osteoclastogenesis is the reason behind various bone pathologies such as osteoporosis, RA, *etc.* Osteoblasts on the other hand are bone-forming ones. Osteoblasts arise from the mesenchymal progenitors that also give rise to adipocytes, chondrocytes, and fibroblasts. Osteoblasts secrete the type 1 collagen that makes 90% of the bone matrix and various extracellular proteins such as osteocalcin and alkaline phosphatase (ALP). Osteoblasts also secrete various growth factors such as insulin-like growth factor (IGF), fibroblast growth factor (FGF), transforming growth factor (TGF), and bone morphogenic protein (BMP) [2]. Osteoblasts express the transcription factor RUNX2 and at matured stages both RANKL and osterix. Bone remodeling is the balancing act between the osteoblasts and the osteoclasts by a phenomenon called coupling. Osteoblasts secrete RANKL which promotes osteoclastogenesis. On the other hand osteoblasts also secrete the osteoprotegerin (OPG) which binds to the RANKL and prevents its binding to the RANK receptor leading to inhibition of osteoclastogenesis. OPG is, therefore, also called as a decoy receptor [5]. The osteoblasts that are entrapped in the bone matrix are called osteocytes. Osteocytes form a network of thin canaliculi that permeates the entire bone matrix and are supposed to provide signals to other osteocytes and osteoblasts. These are also the most abundant and long-lived cells as they can survive for decades in the bone matrix. Osteocytes have a very important role in bone regulation. Osteocytes regulate bone metabolism by regulating both osteoblasts and osteoclasts. Osteocytes produce various signals that induce osteoblastogenesis such as prostaglandin E2, growth factors, glycoproteins, *etc* [6]. Osteocytes negatively regulate the bone by producing the sclerostin protein which acts on the osteoblasts and inhibits bone formation. Sclerostin inhibits the Wnt/B catenin pathway by binding to the low-density lipoprotein receptor-related protein (LRP) 5/6 receptor present on the osteoblast membrane [7]. Osteocytes also secrete RANKL which induces osteoclastogenesis. Proper functioning of our skeletal system requires the critical management of bone remodeling as irregularities in the bone remodeling process result in various skeletal deformities. Several biochemical and mechanical factors such as parathyroid hormone (PTH), estrogen, glucocorticoids, IGF, BMP, TGF-β, *etc.* are involved in the regulation of bone remodeling [8]. Apart from these factors, vitamin D is also a very profound player in bone remodeling. Vitamin D influences the activity of bone cells both directly and indirectly and deficiency of vitamin D leads to skeletal manifestations such as osteoporosis. Recent studies have highlighted the significant role of the immune system in the maintenance of bone metabolism. It is observed that vitamin D has great immunomodulatory potential and prevents various bone pathologies by suppressing the inflammatory environment. However, vitamin D-mediated regulation of bone health by modulating the immune system is not critically revised. Therefore, here we comprehensively discuss the effect of vitamin D on immune system starting with the role of immune system in regulating bone health. Furthermore, we discuss the immunomodulatory potential of vitamin D as a treatment therapy for bone disorders like osteoporosis, RA, and osteoarthritis.

OSTEOIMMUNOLOGY

The term Osteoimmunology was coined for the description of a research field that deals with the interaction between bone and the immune system. Both bone and immune cells share a common origin *i.e.* bone marrow. Immune cells are found to have a very crucial role in regulating bone biology. Findings in the last few years have highlighted the massive breadth of interconnection between bone and immune system and as a result, at present, the role of various immune factors is identified in the maintenance of bone homeostasis. Both innate (monocytes, macrophages, dendritic cells-DCs, innate lymphoid cells-ILCs) and adaptive immune cells (T cells and B cells) are important for maintaining bone homeostasis. Dysregulation in the activity of these immune cells results in several skeletal manifestations. Several studies suggest that the immune system has an immense role in the regulation of bone health under both physiological and pathological conditions and thus novel immune therapies can be designed for the treatment of bone deformities. Vitamin D possesses potent immunomodulatory properties and therefore can act as an immunotherapeutic for the management of various bone disorders. Below, we have discussed the role of vitamin D in regulating bone health by directly influencing the activity of bone health starting with its metabolism. Further, we have discussed the immunomodulatory role of vitamin D and its potential in preventing various inflammatory bone disorders.

VITAMIN D METABOLISM

Vitamin D3 (cholecalciferol) is consumed through dairy products and fish oils in the diet, or it is produced in the skin by UV radiation from 7-dehydrocholesterol. Cholecalciferol is an inactive form of Vitamin D3 and needs to be converted to its biologically active form that influences a wide range of physiological processes [9]. For the same, vitamin D binding protein (DBP) transports vitamin D to the liver through the blood. The enzyme 25-hydroxylase (CYP2R1) in the liver converts vitamin D into the hormone 25-hydroxyvitamin D [$25(OH)D_3$], which is the main form of vitamin D that circulates in the blood [10]. Since a homozygous mutation of the CYP2R1 gene was identified in a patient with low circulating levels of $25(OH)D_3$ and typical signs of vitamin D deficiency, it has been suggested that CYP2R1 is an essential enzyme needed for 25-hydroxylation of vitamin D [11]. Excess non-hydroxylated vitamin D is stored in the liver, adipose tissue, and muscle. $25(OH)D_3$, the primary circulatory form of vitamin D is carried by the DBP to the kidney. In the proximal renal tubule, the biologically active version of the hormone, 1,25 di-hydroxyvitamin D3 [$1,25(OH)_2D_3$] is generated through the degradation of DBP and hydroxylation of $25(OH)D_3$ at position 1 of the A ring by 1α- hydroxylase (CYP27B1) [10]. Even though the kidneys are the primary site for the cytochrome P450 monooxygenase 25(OH)D 1α- hydroxylase [CYP27B1; 1a(OH)ase], it is also present in extrarenal areas like the placenta, monocytes, and macrophages [9]. Fibroblast growth factor–23 (FGF-23) and PTH are both involved in the regulation of CYP27B1 inside the renal tubules. PTH promotes while FGF-23 inhibits 1α-hydroxylase synthesis in the kidney through a series of feedbacks [12]. Vitamin D dependent rickets (VDDR) type 1 is caused by inactivating mutations in the 1a(OH)ase gene despite adequate vitamin D intake, highlighting the significance of the 1a(OH)ase enzyme [9]. Vitamin D metabolites are transported in blood bound to DBP and albumin. Very little vitamin D circulates as free form. Under certain pathological conditions, these transport proteins may be lost. So, even if the free concentrations of vitamin D may be adequate, people with hepatic, intestinal, or renal disorders may have low total levels of vitamin D metabolites without being vitamin D deficient [13, 14].

EFFECTS OF VITAMIN D ON BONE

Vitamin D is the critical player in the regulation of bone heath. Rickets is the primary phenotype of nutritional vitamin D insufficiency, altered vitamin D responsiveness, such as VDR mutations (hereditary vitamin D-resistant rickets), and inadequate $1,25(OH)_2D$ synthesis as a result of CYP27B1 mutations (pseudo-vitamin D deficiency) [15]. According to studies, vitamin D metabolites can alter the responsiveness of bone to growth hormone as well as the expression and/or secretion of many skeletally derived factors. These factors include IGF-1, its receptor and binding proteins, TGF-β, vascular endothelial growth factor (VEGF), interleukin (IL)-6, IL-4, and endothelin receptors, all of which can have an impact on bone on their own and can also influence how vitamin D metabolites affect bone [14]. Vitamin D can also directly influence the activity of bone cells as discussed in the following sections.

Osteoblast

The presence of vitamin D receptor in osteoblasts enables direct effects of $1\alpha,25D_3$ on osteoblasts [16]. In all research works involving human osteoblasts and human mesenchymal stem/stromal cells (MSC), $1,25D_3$ has been found to induce bone formation and mineralization as well as osteogenic differentiation from human MSC [17 - 20]. One finding is that $1,25(OH)_2D_3$ promotes osteoblast development in human marrow stromal cells (hMSCs) *via* CYP27B1/1α-hydroxylase [21]. $1,25D_3$ has also been reported to enhance mineralization by effects on human osteoblasts prior to the onset of mineralization *via* accelerated production of mature matrix vesicles [22].

Although, in contrast to human and rat studies, $1,25D_3$ suppresses differentiation and mineralization in cultures of murine osteoblasts and murine VDR deficient osteoblasts are shown to have increased osteogenic potential [23 - 25]. *In vitro* mineralization has been found to be inhibited by high doses of $1,25D_3$ [26]. On the other hand, $1,25D_3$ has been shown to boost osteoblast mineralization by activating Dickkopf- related-protein- 1 (DKK1) [27]. On the other hand, enhanced bone production and mineralization are shown in transgenic murine models that overexpress the osteoblast specific VDR. In another study, researchers have shown that mice lacking the VDR in osteoblasts have higher bone mass due to lower bone resorption [28]. Another study has revealed that giving ovariectomized rats eldecalcitol, a Vitamin D analogue, on a regular basis reduces bone resorption and induces osteoblast precursors to develop into mature osteoblasts *in vivo* [29]. Together these studies have indicated the contradictory role of vitamin D in osteoblasts regulation.

Osteoclast

In addition to its role in promoting bone formation, $1,25(OH)_2D$ promotes bone resorption by increasing the number and activity of osteoclasts. The effect may be direct where the osteoclast contains VDR and CYP27B1 and 25(OH)D promotes their differentiation in the presence of MCSF and RANKL [30, 31]. According to a research, VDR-mediated activity of $1,25(OH)_2D$ in osteoblasts is necessary to stimulate the osteoclast development [32]. Osteoblasts produce membrane-associated RANKL that activates RANK on osteoclasts and their hematopoietic precursors. This cell-to-cell interaction, together with the MCSF also produces and supports the differentiation of precursors to osteoclasts and enhances their activity. Upstream of the transcription site of the murine and human RANKL gene, several functional vitamin D response elements (VDREs) have been discovered, which potentially make $1,25(OH)_2D_3$ one of the most effective inducers of RANKL expression [33]. A study has indicated that $1\alpha,25\text{-}(OH)_2D_3$ in the presence of MCSF and RANKL increases both the number of osteoclasts and their bone resorption activity during the differentiation of RAW264.7 cells [34]. Another study has verified earlier findings that $1,25(OH)_2D_3$ is a powerful inducer of RANKL expression that accelerates osteoclast-mediated bone resorption in RA [35]. In contrast, few studies have further demonstrated how $1,25(OH)_2D_3$ inhibits the development of arthritis in both RA patients and murine experimental models [36]. According to Kim *et al.* $1,25(OH)_2D_3$ suppresses human osteoclastogenesis and lowers the number of RANK$^+$ osteoclast precursors by down-regulating the activity of the M-CSF receptor c-Fms, which is necessary for the expression of RANK. $1\alpha,25(OH)_2D_3$ is also shown to stimulate the expression of interferon β, an inhibitor of osteoclastogenesis, in osteoclast precursors [37] (Fig. **1**).

Osteocyte

In contrast to the vast knowledge about vitamin D target genes in osteoblasts, less is known about the specific vitamin D-responsive genes in osteocytes. It has been demonstrated that $1,25(OH)_2D_3$ enhances the transcription of RANKL, BMP7 and FGF23 in osteocytes or osteocyte-like cells [38 - 40]. RANKL is one of the master regulators of osteoclastic bone resorption. Moreover, based on what is known about osteoblasts, $1,25(OH)_2D_3$ is likely to be responsible for regulating the mRNA abundance of genes involved in mineralization, including progressive ankylosis, osteocalcin, osteopontin, ectonucleotide pyrophosphatase/phospho-diesterase 1 (Enpp1), and Enpp3 in osteocytes [41]. In addition, $1,25(OH)_2D_3$ may upregulate osteoclastic bone resorption and restrict bone mineralization in osteocyte lacunae by increasing RANKL expression. It is reported that vitamin D plays a role in the regulation of osteocyte number and perilacunar remodeling in both human and murine models. It's interesting to note that in osteocyte cultures, $1,25(OH)_2D_3$ has recently been shown to promote mineralization and regulate key genes linked to mineral regulation, including Fgf23 and dentin matrix acidic phosphoprotein 1 (Dmp) in differentiated IDG-SW3 osteocyte-like cells [42]. The loss of these regulatory functions is caused by the selective deletion of the VDR in mouse osteocytes, indicating that the osteocyte is a distinct target of $1,25(OH)_2D_3$ activity *in vivo* [43].

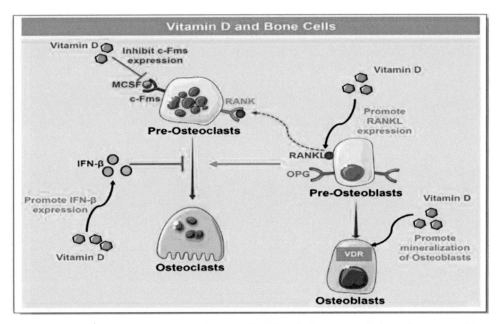

Fig. (1). Vitamin D regulates the activity of bone cells. Vitamin D treatment induces the pre-osteoblasts to express RANKL which binds the RANK receptor present on pre-osteoclasts and thereby promotes osteoclastogenesis. In another mechanism, vitamin D inhibits osteoclastogenesis by inhibiting expression of c-Fms which is a receptor for MCSF, and induces expression of IFN-β which suppresses osteoclast formation. Vitamin D also promotes mineralization of osteoblasts and thus promotes bone formation.

IMMUNOMODULATORY ROLE OF VITAMIN D

Immune cells play a significant role in maintaining the control of inflammatory response, and bone remodeling. Beyond maintaining calcium and bone health, vitamin D also plays a crucial role in the regulation of innate and adaptive immune responses, as well as in the prevention of autoimmune disorders. Arora *et al.* (2022) have reported that the presence of Vitamin D receptors on the immune cells like B cells, T cells, innate lymphoid cells (ILCs), and macrophages play a major role in the development and function of the immune system [44]. The complicated regulation of vitamin VDR expression in immune cells based on their matching activation status serves as an example of the complex interaction between vitamin D and immune cells. Additionally, CYP27B1 and CYP24A1 expression suggests that immune system cells have the potential to tightly control the availability and efficacy of the active metabolite of vitamin D [44]. In the present section, we go over how vitamin D affects these immune cells, which are crucial in the development of infectious and autoimmune illnesses (Table **1**).

EFFECTS OF VITAMIN D ON INNATE IMMUNE SYSTEM

The innate immune system is the primary line of defence against various infections and must act quickly to combat encroaching invaders. Innate immune system recognizes elements from both the host and local microorganisms. It comprises physical defense against infection *via* skin, mucus, and vascular endothelial cells. Along with these, there are phagocytic cells, antimicrobial proteins, and cells (such as dendritic cells, macrophages, natural killer, and neutrophil cells). Vitamin D has been reported to regulate the innate immune system by improving the phagocytic capacity [45] and promoting physical barrier functions [46, 47].

Monocytes/Macrophages

Monocytes and macrophages contribute significantly to the defense against infections by releasing cytokines. Toll-like receptors (TLRs) found on the surfaces of these cells identify components from bacteria, viruses, and fungi, which upregulate the expression of the VDR and CYP27B1. CYP27B1 is responsible for the metabolism of vitamin D which converts it into the active form, 1,25D. This leads to enhanced production of antimicrobial peptides, which act by assisting in the rupturing of cell membranes of pathogens or by initiating an antibiotic signaling cascade in infected cells. In a study it has been reported that vitamin D acts as an inflammation suppressor. It was found that human monocytes and bone marrow-derived macrophages (BMM) from mice expressed considerably more mitogen-activated protein kinase phosphatase-1 (MKP-1) after vitamin D treatment, blocking the production of pro-inflammatory cytokines from monocyte/macrophage [48]. Also, vitamin D3 therapy has been demonstrated to reduce the expression of TLR2 and TLR4 in monocytes, as well as pro-inflammatory cytokines, chemokines, and monocyte trafficking [48]. Another study has demonstrated that during the development of macrophages, 1,25D upregulates the production of the complement receptor immunoglobulin (CRIg), which is responsible for enhanced phagocytosis in bacterial and fungal infections [49]. These results imply that macrophages have an intrinsic defense system that is vitamin D-primed. It is also found that 1,25D by increasing glutathione reductase (GR) and glutamate-cysteine ligase (GCL) exerts an anti-oxidative effect on monocytes. This reduces the production of oxygen radicals (like reactive oxygen species)(ROS) [48, 49]. Hence, highlighting the anti-oxidative effect on monocytes, it has been demonstrated that vitamin D could change the epigenome of immune cells, specifically monocytes, and the differentiated phenotypes they give rise to macrophages. Therefore, when monocytes differentiate into either macrophages or dendritic cells, they stop expressing VDR.

Dendritic Cells

Dendritic cells bridge the gap between innate and adaptive immune responses, and they are essential in determining how the adaptive immune response develops. Vitamin D is responsible for regulating the maturation of dendritic cells. Several studies have indicated the tolerogenic effect of vitamin D3 on dendritic cells [50, 51]. This is found to be facilitated by metabolic reprogramming that is *via* affecting biological pathways majorly including the tricarboxylic acid cycle (TCA), mitochondrial electron transport, and electron transport chain (ETC). In a recent study, it has been reported that the exposure of dendritic cells to vitamin D3 inhibits neutrophil-dependent stimulation of dendritic cells which drives Th17 cell generation from naïve T cells and also promotes Treg cell formation [52]. This supports the use of vitamin D3 to treat inflammatory disorders or autoimmune illnesses in dendritic cells targeting vaccines [53]. Another study has indicated the role of calcitriol in decreasing the transfer of viral particles from dendritic cells to CD4$^+$T cells by down regulating the expression of receptors responsible for the transfer of virus, hence lowering the percentage of infected cells in human immunodeficiency virus (HIV) infection. Saul *et al.* (2019) have demonstrated that the ineffective priming of T cells by $1,25(OH)_2D_3$ conditioned bone marrow-derived dendritic cells (BMDC) is not only attributable to the down-regulated expression of major histocompatibility complex (MHC) class II and co-stimulatory molecules like CD40, CD80, and CD86 [54, 55]. The ability of BMDC to stimulate T cells is further constrained by the activation of inhibitory pathways that occurs when $1,25(OH)_2D3$ is exposed to BMDC during development [56, 57] (Fig. **2**).

Vitamin D has been found to regulate early cytokine generation by ILCs in the gut thereby making it useful in preventing enteric infections. It has been proven that the vitamin D/VDR signaling pathway plays a crucial role in controlling ILC3 growth in mice's guts through the production of IL-22, which offers strong innate immunity against *C. rodentium* infection [58, 59]. Interestingly, vitamin D_3 is found to prevent human ILCs from expressing gut-homing integrin and producing various effector cytokines that are triggered by RA. Since ILC2s promote allergic inflammation, blocking them with vitamin D3 may lessen allergic inflammation and potentially help in preventing allergic illness [60, 61]. This along with other evidence highlights the antagonist effects of vitamin D and vitamin A in ILCs [62]. Also, vitamin D deficiency is found to be a risk factor for inflammatory bowel disease (IBD) and targeting IL-23/12 is a promising strategy in the treatment of IBD. The IL-23-driven tissue resident group 3 ILCs (ILC3s) perform critical functions in intestinal immunity, proposing a fresh mechanism for controlling intestinal inflammation by manipulating ILC3s [63, 64]. A study done by Ercolano *et al.* (2022) has reported that the supplementation of vitamin D can be an intriguing therapeutic strategy to reduce IFN-γ mediated ILC precursors (ILCP) release, as high levels of IFN-γ in the celiac disease cytokine profile are accompanied by an increase in ILC precursors (ILCPs) [65].

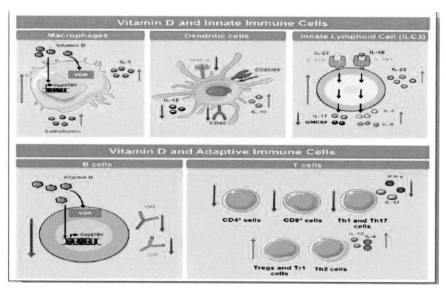

Fig. (2). Effect of vitamin D on both innate and adaptive immune cells. Vitamin D promotes the innate immune cells such as macrophages, dendritic cells and ILC3 through several mechanisms. Vitamin D downregulates IgG and IgM production from B cells and stimulates the activity of anti-inflammatory T cells such as Tregs while downregulating the activity of inflammatory T cells like Th17 cells.

EFFECTS OF VITAMIN D ON THE ADAPTIVE IMMUNE SYSTEM

Adaptive immunity which includes both cell-mediated and humoral immunity targets primarily invasive infections. After an initial encounter with a particular pathogen, immunological memory is developed which results in an improved response to subsequent encounters with the same pathogen through magnified production of neutralizing antibodies. In addition to the activating role of vitamin D on the innate immune system to improve the rapid response to infection, vitamin D also exerts a profound effect on the adaptive immune system. According to exploratory studies, vitamin D causes adaptive immune system cells to adopt a more tolerogenic state, which may be used to treat autoimmune illnesses. Up to 500 gene expression is regulated when $1,25(OH)_2D_3$ binds to the intracellular VDR. It has been demonstrated that in contrast to resting monocytes and dendritic cells which have intracellular VDR expression, resting T and B lymphocytes exhibit minimal to negligible VDR expression, but in response to this, VDR expression increases [66]. In further sections, we will discuss vitamin D's role in modulating adaptive immune response subsets.

T cells

T cells are essential adaptive immune system mediators that are regulated by vitamin D particularly $1,25(OH)_2D_3$ in both direct as well as indirect manner [66, 67]. The direct effect of vitamin D3 is more controversial because it is dependent on the activation status of T cells, as it has been found that upon activation, the VDR increases. Vitamin D polarizes T cells to a regulatory and anti-inflammatory profile *via* its modulating effects on the transcription factors of these cells [68]. The cytokine expression can be suppressed by VDR/retinoid-X-receptor (RXR) heterodimers which are formed in the presence of $1,25(OH)_2D_3$ and lead to the displacement of DNA-bound nuclear factor (NF-AT). It is observed that in bone disorders, regulatory T cells (Tregs) are either deficient or become impaired. Tregs are reported to suppress osteoclastogenesis mainly in a cell-to-cell contact-dependent manner *via* cytotoxic T lymphocyte-associated antigen (CTLA)-4 and in part by secretion of TGF-β, interleukin (IL)-10, and IL-4 [69]. CTLA-4 binds to the CD80/86 present on osteoclast precursors inhibiting their suppression. However, Kim *et al.*, reported that IL-4 and TGF-β are key molecules involved in the inhibition of osteoclastogenesis by Tregs and not in a cell-cell contact dependent manner [70]. Luo *et al.* have shown that Tregs inhibit osteo-clastogenesis in both human peripheral blood mononuclear cells (PBMCs) and bone marrow cells in an IL-10 and TGF-β-dependent manner. The addition of anti-IL-10 and anti-TGF-β antibodies completely blocks the inhibition of osteoclastogenesis by Tregs [71]. In contrast to the previously reported studies, recently a study has reported that Tregs induced by IL-1β can lead to bone erosion. IL-1β-induced Tregs show an aberrant expression of RANKL which mediates RANKL-induced osteoclastogenesis [72]. Tregs express transcription factor forkhead box P3 (FOXP3) which is found to be upregulated in the presence of vitamin D_3 [73]. It is reported that vitamin D3 inhibits T-cell proliferation. $1,25(OH)_2D_3$ suppresses the synthesis of Th1 cytokines (such as IFN-γ, IL-2) *via* JAK/STAT pathway [74], Th9 cytokines, and Th17 cytokines (such as IL-21) and hence proven to be responsible for inducing self-tolerance. Also these cells are found to have a relatively high expression of VDR as compared to others [67, 75, 76]. The indirect way involves altering the capacity of antigen-presenting cells (APCs) to stimulate T lymphocytes. As discussed earlier $1,25(OH)_2D_3$ lowers the expression of class II MHC and other co-stimulatory molecules (like CD40, CD80, and CD86) on the surface of monocytes as well as macrophages, thereby resulting in reduced antigen presentation. $1,25(OH)_2VD_3$ was also observed to increase the differentiation of Tregs indirectly by affecting VDR/Phospholipase C-γ1 (PLC-γ1)/ TGF-β pathway which induces FOXP3 [77]. According to a few recent studies, which assessed the effect of vitamin D3 in allergic as well as inflammatory conditions, it was observed that the administration of vitamin D3 significantly decreased Th2 and Th17 while increasing Th1 and Tregs [78, 79]. This clearly shows that vitamin D3 can prevent and treat allergic rhinitis, but another study couldn't confirm this [80]. Contradicting to this it is also being reported that vitamin D3 inhibits type 1 T cells secretion which promotes wound healing in diabetic foot ulcers (DFU), which are associated with vitamin D deficiency. Hence the investigation on a large scale has reported that DFU may be avoided by increasing $1,25(OH)_2D_3$ levels through dietary supplements in Diabetic Mellitus patients [81].

There have been few investigations into the impact of $1,25(OH)_2D_3$ on CD8$^+$ T cells, hence little is known. The proliferation of CD8$^+$ T cells may be prevented, unaffected, or even boosted in the presence of several stimuli due to $1,25(OH)_2D_3$ [82, 83]. There are only a few studies indicating the direct effect of vitamin D on CD8$^+$ T cells. A study on patients with multiple sclerosis shows that CD8$^+$ T cells respond to vitamin D directly, modulating their immune system [84, 85]. An another study using the well-known VDR gene ablation mouse model of infection with pathogens, has uncovered the role of $1,25(OH)_2D_3$ signaling in regulating CD8$^+$ T cell differentiation during infection. This study has also investigated the altered production of chemokine receptors and chemokines as well. $1,25(OH)_2D_3$ is expected to control CD69 mediated sphinosine-1-phosphate receptor subtype-1 (S1P1) expression as in the absence of $1,25(OH)_2D_3$ it leads to enhanced lymph node localization of CD8$^+$ T cells [86]. Vitamin D is also reported to be a regulatory agent for tumor growth followed by CD8$^+$ T cells infiltration, which can be a potential adjuvant for treating breast malignancies as this proves to facilitate a better prognosis [87].

B CELLS

The presence of VDR in active B lymphocytes indicates that vitamin D has a significant impact on B-lymphocyte function. B cells were shown to express CYP27b1, suggesting that they may be able to produce autocrine or intracrine reactions towards vitamin D [88].

Vitamin D's effects on adaptive immunity include a reduction in B cell development and proliferation [89]. Vitamin D deficiency is a pivotal factor for the systemic lupus erythematosus (SLE) suggested by the fact that vitamin D3 absence is linked to increased immunoglobin synthesis, as well as an increase in the number of memory B cells [90]. Therefore, it is appealing to hypothesize that a lower level of 1,25 $(OH)_2D_3$ may have an aggravating function in the pathogenesis of SLE by releasing a physiological brake on humoral immunity. It has been proposed that the impact of 1,25$(OH)_2D_3$ on B cells may be indirectly mediated by its impact on T-cell and/or APC activity. But there are conflicting studies as well which report that the presence of VDR on B cells might be linked to a direct effect [91]. Recently, our group has reported that a subset of B cells *i.e.,* regulatory B cells (Bregs) suppressed osteoclastogenesis in an IL-10 dependent manner. In addition, our group has reported that a reduction in the percentage of Bregs augments bone loss in the preclinical model of osteoporosis [92]. However, the role of vitamin D in the differentiation of Bregs has not been investigated in detail. There is a need to explore more in this context in order to establish a clear role of vitamin D in B cells thus, opening the novel future avenues for research.

Table 1. Role of Vitamin D on Immune Cells.

S. No.	Immune cells	Effect of Vitamin D
1	Monocytes and Macrophages	• Stimulates monocyte proliferation • Increase in IL-1, and cathelicidin (an antimicrobial peptide) synthesis by macrophages. • Enhanced innate immune response.
2	Dendritic Cells	• Inhibit DC maturation • Prevent expression of CD40, CD80, CD86, and MHC class II.
3	Innate Lymphoid Cells (ILCs)	• Decrease ILC2 proliferation . • An essential role in the development of ILC3. • Decrease the synthesis of IFNγ mediated ILC precursors. • Inhibit expression of gut-homing integrin in ILCs. • Decrease the expression of IL-23. pathway-associated cytokines such as IL-17 and GM-CSF in ILC3. • Increase the expression of cytokines associated with the IL-1β pathway such as IL-6 and IL-8.
4	T cells	• Reduce the expression of IL-2, IL-17, and IFN-γ • Decrease CD4$^+$ and CD8$^+$ T lymphocytes. • Stimulate FOXP3 expression thereby promoting Treg cells • Inhibits Th9 & Th17 cell differentiation
5	B cells	• Restrict the development of immunoglobulins • Decrease plasma cell differentiation • Decrease B cell proliferation

TARGETING THE IMMUNOMODULATORY ROLE OF VITAMIN D FOR THE MANAGEMENT OF VARIOUS BONE PATHOLOGIES

As discussed above, vitamin D regulates the activity of a wide range of immune cells and therefore has a role in the prevention of various autoimmune disorders. Therefore, in several bone pathologies, vitamin D is targeted as an immunotherapeutic for the management of inflammatory bone loss as detailed below (Fig. **3**).

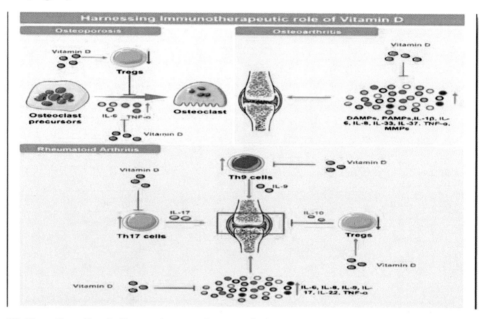

Fig. (3). Targeting vitamin D as an immunotherapeutic for the treatment of bone pathologies. Vitamin D attenuates osteoporosis by inducing Tregs and inhibiting the expression of osteoclastogenic cytokines IL-6 and TNF-α. Immune cells such as Th9, Th17 and cytokines like IL-6, IL-8, IL-9, IL-17, IL-22, TNF-α enhance the pathogenesis of rheumatoid arthritis. Vitamin D administration decreases the level of Th9, Th17 cells and inflammatory cytokines along with simultaneously inducing the differentiation of Tregs and therefore prevents RA. In osteoarthritis, there is an increase in the level of IL-6, IL-8, IL-17, IL-1β, TNF-α, DAMPs, PAMPs and MMPs which lead to cartilage destruction. Treatment with vitamin D further decreases the level of these cytokines and therefore attenuates osteoarthritis.

Vitamin D and Osteoporosis

Osteoporosis is a bone deformity that leads to low bone mineral density and decreased bone strength. Osteoporosis is often called as a "silent disease" as it remains undiagnosed until a fracture occurs. It is one of the most common inflammatory bone disorders affecting the lives of more than 200 million people worldwide. In recent years, various therapeutic modulations are exploited for the treatment of osteoporosis such as bisphosphonates, denosumab, estrogen replacement therapies and parathyroid hormone analogies [93]. Vitamin D is an important factor in the regulation of bone health and several studies have shown that vitamin D supplementation prevents bone loss. It has a critical impact on reducing the fracture risk. A meta-analysis has shown that vitamin D along with calcium has decreased the risk of fractures [94]. Daily intake of calcium and vitamin D enriched milk is able to increase the BMD of femoral neck in postmenopausal healthy women [95]. Vitamin D supplementation has also been able to prevent partial bone loss in ovariectomized mice with significant bone microstructure improvement of mandibular condyle [96]. However, there are studies that have shown that a high dose of vitamin D is associated with adverse side effects, especially in females and therefore its use should be carefully recommended [97]. Vitamin D stimulates the absorption of calcium and phosphate by opening the calcium channels in intestine and inducing the formation of calcium binding proteins in intestinal cells. Vitamin D deficiency therefore decreases the mineralization process and thus induces bone loss [98]. Vitamin D analogue eldecalcitol in combination with hypoglycemic drug exendin-4 has been observed to prevent the diabetic osteoporosis. Eldecalcitol attenuates osteoporosis by decreasing both the formation and function of osteoclasts *via* increasing the EphrinB2-EphB4 signaling between osteoclasts and osteoblasts [99]. Immune system has a very vast role in the regulation of bone health as we have already discussed above, and osteoporosis is a result of immune dysregulation. Immune cells are pivotal players in the pathophysiology of osteoporosis as emphasized by several studies. Immune cells mediated inflammation is the major contributor to the pathogenesis of post-menopausal osteoporosis (PMO). Inflammatory cytokines produced by immune cells, especially T cells tip the balance in favor of bone resorption *via* promoting osteoclastogenesis [100]. The role of Tregs-Th17 cell axis is well established in the context of PMO by our group [101 - 103] and now the role of other immune cells is also being unraveled. It is observed that a regulatory subset of B cells *i.e.* Bregs also interweaves the bone and immune system and are very crucial in maintaining skeletal homeostasis. Bregs are protective against bone loss and inhibit osteoclastogenesis *via* producing IL-10. PMO mice model has significantly reduced frequency of $CD19^+IL-10^+$ Bregs and $CD19^+CD1d^{hi}CD5^+IL-10^+$ "B10" Bregs as compared to sham mice. Moreover, ovx mice has significantly lower level of IL-10 in serum as compared to sham mice [92]. This cross talk or close association of bone and immune cells in the prevention or pathogenesis of osteoporosis gives birth to a new field of biology named by our group as "Immunoporosis"(*i.e.* immunology of osteoporosis) that specifically deals with the role of immune cells in osteoporosis [104 - 106]. It is observed that the immunomodulatory potential of vitamin D is also utilized in the treatment of osteoporosis apart from its usual role in bone mineralization. It is reported that eldecalcitol in combination with exendin-4 synergistically induces osteogenic differentiation of bone marrow stromal cells *via* inducing M2 macrophages polarization [107]. Post-menopausal women with osteoporosis have increased concentration of inflammatory cytokines IL-6 and TNF-α. Vitamin D treatment along with calcium significantly decreases the level of these inflammatory cytokines [108]. Vitamin D administration increases the frequency of Tregs and foxp3 expression in the PMO mice model [109]. Thus, vitamin D can be a novel immune approach in the management of osteoporosis.

Vitamin D and Rheumatoid Arthritis

RA is a chronic systemic autoimmune disorder that affects the joints resulting in the destruction of the cartilage of joints and weakening of the tendons and ligaments [110]. It is the result of severe inflammatory responses such as an increase in the level of pathogenic Th17 cells and inflammatory cytokines. It has been observed that Vitamin D deficiency is common in RA patients and is a risk factor for RA [111]. A significant inverse correlation exists between vitamin D and all-cause mortality rate due to RA [112]. Vitamin D deficiency in RA patients indicates a more severe and active disease and can be used to predict the disability, disease activity, and radiographic damage over the first year of the disease [113, 114]. RA patients which are rheumatoid factor (RF) positive have more chances to be vitamin D-deficient as compared to those with RF negative and, therefore, vitamin D levels in RA patients can be correlated with the disease severity [115]. It is reported that weekly supplementation of 60,000 IU of vitamin D3 to RA patients provides greater pain relief [116]. Other studies also utilize vitamin D therapy for arthritis. It is observed that nano-encapsulations consisting of a combination of curcumin and vitamin D3 successfully inhibit the inflammation and myeloperoxidase (MPO) activity in the mice model of arthritis [117].

The major mechanism through which vitamin D supplementation reduces the severity of RA is *via* regulation of the immune system. Vitamin D acts on synovial fibroblasts (SF) which have an important role in the pathogenesis of RA. *In vitro* cultures of SFs from the RA patients show a higher expression of NOD-, LRR- and pyrin containing domain 3 (NLRP3) inflammasome which is found to be positively correlated with the level of anti-cyclic citrullinated peptide (CCP), RF, and C-reactive protein (CRP). However, the treatment of SFs with vitamin D downregulates the expression of the NLRP3, TLR1, and TLR4 thus highlighting the potential anti-inflammatory response of vitamin D [118]. Another study has reported that arthritis gets exaggerated in mice fed with the vitamin D deficient conditions. However, supplementation of diet sufficient in vitamin D attenuates arthritis. Vitamin D prevents the inflammatory conditions induced during arthritis by inhibiting inflammatory cytokines from T cells. Strikingly vitamin D also upregulates the expression of the leukocyte associated Vitamin D supplementation with anti-rheumatic drugs like tocilizumab, which not only induces the development of Tregs but also inhibits the differentiation of Th17 cells and subsequent release of IL-17 [123]. In case of autoimmune diseases like RA, the activity of various memory T cells gets elevated. These cells express C-C motif chemokine receptor 6 (CCR6) and RORC and release various inflammatory cytokines such as IL-17A, IFN-γ, and TNF-α. It is observed that vitamin D treatment of these memory Th cells that are isolated from the RA patients inhibits the secretion of inflammatory cytokines from these cells with an accompanied expression of various anti-inflammatory cytokines such as IL-10 and CTLA-4. Strikingly, these vitamin D-induced cells can migrate to the inflammatory milieu and suppress the autologous CD3$^+$ Tcells just like the Tregs. Therefore, vitamin D has great immunomodulatory potential and can convert a pathogenic subtype of the immune cell into the non-pathogenic one [124]. Similar results have also been shown by another study in which it is observed that Vitamin D treatment decreases the incidence and arthritis score in the CIA mice model by downregulating the number of Th17 cells while promoting the development of Tregs. Vitamin D treatment decreases the differentiation of Th17 cells by downregulation of the IL-6R expression and its downstream signaling in an miR-124 dependent manner. The use of the miR-124 inhibitor reverses the effect of vitamin D on Th17 cell differentiation [125]. Vitamin D supplementation is also observed to prevent the secretion of inflammatory cytokines such as IFN-γ, IL-17, IL-6, TNF-α, and IL-22 while upregulating the expression of IL-4 and therefore modulating the level of cytokines to prevent arthritis [126]. In continuity with this, another study has shown that vitamin D and dexamethasone additively inhibit the secretion of inflammatory cytokines such as INF-γ, IL-17, and IL-22 from the CCR6$^+$ memory Th cells and IL-6, and IL-8 from the RA synovial fibroblasts [124]. Vitamin D treatments *in vitro* have been found to inhibit the IL-22-mediated osteoclast fibroblast-like synoviocytes isolated from RA patients by suppressing the RANKL expression *via* regulating the Janus kinase-2/signal transducers and activators of transcription-3 (JAK-2/STAT-3) or p38 mitogen activated protein kinase (MAPK)/NF-κB signaling pathway [127]. Therefore, it can be concluded that vitamin D supplementation along with the right levels of anti-rheumatic dugs can be beneficial in decreasing the severity of RA by diminishing the inflammatory responses.

Vitamin D and Osteoarthritis

Osteoarthritis [OA] is a musculoskeletal disorder which affects the joints preferentially the hip, knee, and spine joints. Approximately 250 million people around the globe are suffering from OA [128]. Although various factors are involved in the pathogenesis of OA, but immune system is the peculiar one.

Various inflammatory cytokines such as TNF-α, IL-1β, TLR2 and 4, complement proteins like C5, damage associated molecular patterns (DAMPs) and pathogen-associated molecular patterns (PAMPs) participate in the cascade of reactions that induce the degradation of cartilage matrix resulting in the progression of OA [129]. Several studies have supported that vitamin D can mitigate osteoarthritis. OA patients have significantly lower levels of Vitamin D in the serum highlighting the possibility that vitamin D has a role in the pathogenesis of OA [130]. Vitamin D levels have been observed to be decreased in a significant number of OA patients and vitamin D deficiency is strongly correlated with disability, pain intensity, anxiety, functional impairment, walking speed, and hesitancy in social participation [131]. It is observed that patients with decreased vitamin D levels are mainly in stages III and IV of OA [132]. In continuity with this, Montemor *et al.* have also reported that patients with vitamin D deficiency have a higher disease index with increased clinical disease severity and functional impairment as compared to patients with normal vitamin D levels [133]. Several other studies have supported that vitamin D deficiency contributes majorly to the severity of osteoarthritis. Therefore, vitamin D can be an early prognostic marker in the diagnosis of OA. Vitamin D supplementation on the other hand is reported to improve the knee architecture in OA patients [134]. The major mechanism through which vitamin D attenuates OA is by suppressing the inflammation. It is reported that Vitamin D deficiency enhances cartilage degradation by upregulating the expression of various inflammatory markers like TLRs, TNF-a, IL-33, IL-37, MMPs, and DAMPs resulting in the development of osteoarthritis. However, the supplementation of vitamin D restores the level of these markers and induces the polarization of macrophages towards the anti-inflammatory M2 type which further dampens the inflammation and thus supporting cartilage synthesis [135]. Vitamin D also regulates the level of macrophage migration inhibitory factor (MIR) which might have a role in the progression of OA [132]. In knee osteoarthritis, patients' vitamin D status has been found to be inversely correlated with the expression of inflammatory markers. Knee OA patients with low vitamin D status have higher levels of inflammatory markers such as IL-1β, TNF-α, hs-CRP, and NF-κB p65 whereas that with high vitamin D status have a lower expression of inflammatory markers suggesting that vitamin D is inversely associated with inflammation [136]. Moreover, vitamin D supplementation is able to control the disease severity of OA by regulating the IL-6 level [137]. Vitamin D also induces the autophagy in the chondrocytes by regulating the AMP-activated protein kinase (AMPK)-mammalian target of rapamycin (mTOR) signaling pathway which reduces the secretion of TNF-α and IL-6 from both cartilage tissue and chondrocytes [138]. Another factor that could play a role in vitamin D deficiency-mediated pathogenesis of OA is the gut microbiota. Gut microbiota has an immense effect on the immune system. Alterations in the gut microbiota composition are associated with inflammation. Thus, there can be a possibility that altered gut microbiota under vitamin D deficiency might initiate the progression of OA by inducing the inflammatory conditions. Studies discussed above highlight that vitamin D has an imperative role in OA severity. However, some studies have shown that there is no correlation between vitamin D deficiency and OA [139] and completely neglect the fact that vitamin D is associated with OA [140]. Therefore, there are mixed results on the effect of vitamin D in case of OA. According to a met-analysis on vitamin D's effect on symptomatic and structural outcomes in the case of knee OA, vitamin D administration can decrease the pain but not improve the structural progression of knee OA patients [141]. Various factors play a role in determining the effect of vitamin D in the pathogenesis of OA such as sex. It is observed that vitamin D deficiency is positively correlated with the risk of OA in older men but not in older women [142]. Therefore, based on above discussion it can be concluded that vitamin D supplementation reduces the OA disease symptoms mainly by modulating the immune system. However, several other factors come into play in determining the effect of vitamin D on OA.

CONCLUSION

Vitamin D supplementation has been observed to significantly decrease the bone turnover and fracture risk. All types of bone cells *i.e.* osteoclasts, osteoblasts and osteocytes express VDR and therefore vitamin D can directly regulate the skeletal system. However, the in-depth mechanisms behind the vitamin D mediated regulation of bone health are still not completely unraveled. Recently it is becoming clear that vitamin D also has a profound effect on the immune system apart from its classic effect on the calcium homeostasis as most of the immune cells express VDR. Vitamin D maintains the local immunological milieu by regulating the activity of various adaptive and innate immune cells and its deficiency is found to be associated with increased autoimmunity. Notably recent discoveries have emphasized that a massive scope of communication exists between the bone and the immune system. Fascinating research in the field of osteoimmunology has provided new etiologic paradigms for skeletal disorders and reveals various aspects of dynamic interaction between the skeleton and the immune system. As the immune system is the major player in the regulation of bone health, it is reasonable to think that vitamin D supplementation can prevent bone loss by modulating the immune system. Therefore, it is important to discuss the vitamin D-mediated regulation of bone health in an immune system dependent manner. This will surely help in considering vitamin D as an immune adjuvant therapy with huge clinical implications in the future for the management of inflammatory bone loss in various bone pathologies. However, various facets of immune-mediated regulation of bone health *via* vitamin D are still unknown and thus dedicated research is warranted in the field.

ACKNOWLEDGEMENTS

This work is financially supported by projects: DBT (BT-2189), Govt. of India, and intramural grant (AC-21) sanctioned to RKS. AB, TS, SD, LS and RKS acknowledge the Department of Biotechnology, AIIMS, New Delhi-India for providing infrastructural facilities. AB thanks ICMR for research fellowship. LS thanks the UGC for research fellowship. Figures are created with the help of Servier Medical Art, provided by Servier, licensed under a Creative Commons Attribution 3.0 unported license (https://smart.servier.com).

REFERENCES

[1]   Florencio-Silva R, Sasso GRS, Sasso-Cerri E, Simões MJ, Cerri PS. Biology of bone tissue: Structure, function, and factors that influence bone cells. BioMed Res Int 2015; 2015: 1-17.
        [http://dx.doi.org/10.1155/2015/421746] [PMID: 26247020]

[2]   Hadjidakis DJ, Androulakis II. Bone remodeling.Annals of the New York Academy of Sciences. Blackwell Publishing Inc 2006; pp. 385-96.

[3]   Clarke B. Normal bone anatomy and physiology. Clin J Am Soc Nephrol 2008; 3(Suppl 3) (3): S131-9.
        [http://dx.doi.org/10.2215/CJN.04151206] [PMID: 18988698]

[4]   Boyce B, Yao Z, Xing L. Osteoclasts have multiple roles in bone in addition to bone resorption. Crit Rev Eukaryot Gene Expr 2009; 19(3): 171-80.
        [http://dx.doi.org/10.1615/CritRevEukarGeneExpr.v19.i3.10] [PMID: 19883363]

[5]   Boyle WJ, Simonet WS, Lacey DL. Osteoclast differentiation and activation. Nature 2003; 423(6937): 337-42.
        [http://dx.doi.org/10.1038/nature01658] [PMID: 12748652]

[6]   Robling AG, Bonewald LF. The Osteocyte: New Insights. Annu Rev Physiol 2020; 82(1): 485-506.
        [http://dx.doi.org/10.1146/annurev-physiol-021119-034332] [PMID: 32040934]

[7]   Compton JT, Lee FY. A review of osteocyte function and the emerging importance of sclerostin. J Bone Joint Surg Am 2014; 96(19): 1659-68.
        [http://dx.doi.org/10.2106/JBJS.M.01096] [PMID: 25274791]

[8]   Bhardwaj A, Sapra L, Tiwari A, Mishra PK, Sharma S, Srivastava RK. "Osteomicrobiology": The nexus between bone and bugs. Front Microbiol 2022; 12: 812466.
        [http://dx.doi.org/10.3389/fmicb.2021.812466] [PMID: 35145499]

[9]   Christakos S, Ajibade DV, Dhawan P, Fechner AJ, Mady LJ, Vitamin D. Vitamin D: Metabolism. Rheum Dis Clin North Am 2012; 38(1): 1-11. 1.
        [http://dx.doi.org/10.1016/j.rdc.2012.03.003] [PMID: 22525839]

[10]   Bikle. Genetic Alteration NIH Public Access. Bone 2008; 23: 1-7.

[11]   Cheng JB, Levine MA, Bell NH, Mangelsdorf DJ, Russell DW. Genetic evidence that the human CYP2R1 enzyme is a key vitamin D 25-hydroxylase. Proc Natl Acad Sci 2004; 101(20): 7711-5.
        [http://dx.doi.org/10.1073/pnas.0402490101] [PMID: 15128933]

[12]   Latic N, Erben RG. FGF23 and Vitamin D metabolism. JBMR Plus 2021; 5(12): e10558.
        [http://dx.doi.org/10.1002/jbm4.10558] [PMID: 34950827]

[13]   Bouillon R, Schuit F, Antonio L, Rastinejad F, Vitamin D. Vitamin D binding protein: A historic overview. Front Endocrinol 2020; 10: 910.
[http://dx.doi.org/10.3389/fendo.2019.00910] [PMID: 31998239]

[14]   Bikle DD. Vitamin D and bone. Curr Osteoporos Rep 2012; 10(2): 151-9.
[http://dx.doi.org/10.1007/s11914-012-0098-z] [PMID: 22544628]

[15]   Malloy PJ, Feldman D. Genetic disorders and defects in vitamin D action. Rheum Dis Clin North Am 2012; 38(1): 93-106.
[http://dx.doi.org/10.1016/j.rdc.2012.03.009] [PMID: 22525845]

[16]   van Driel M, van Leeuwen JPTM. Vitamin D endocrine system and osteoblasts. Bonekey Rep 2014; 3: 493.
[http://dx.doi.org/10.1038/bonekey.2013.227] [PMID: 24605210]

[17]   Zhou S, Glowacki J, Kim SW, *et al.* Clinical characteristics influence *in vitro* action of 1,25-dihydroxyvitamin D $_3$ in human marrow stromal cells. J Bone Miner Res 2012; 27(9): 1992-2000.
[http://dx.doi.org/10.1002/jbmr.1655] [PMID: 22576852]

[18]   al L et. ©. Chinese Medical Association Publishing House Downloaded from medCentral.net on (February 24, 2022). For personal use only Med Assoc Publ house 2011; 35-44.

[19]   Jørgensen NR, Henriksen Z, Sørensen OH, Civitelli R. Dexamethasone, BMP-2, and 1,25-dihydroxyvitamin D enhance a more differentiated osteoblast phenotype: Validation of an *in vitro* model for human bone marrow-derived primary osteoblasts. Steroids 2004; 69(4): 219-26.
[http://dx.doi.org/10.1016/j.steroids.2003.12.005] [PMID: 15183687]

[20]   Prince M, Banerjee C, Javed A, *et al.* Expression and regulation of Runx2/Cbfa1 and osteoblast phenotypic markers during the growth and differentiation of human osteoblasts. J Cell Biochem 2001; 80(3): 424-40.
[http://dx.doi.org/10.1002/1097-4644(20010301)80:3<424::AID-JCB160>3.0.CO;2-6]   [PMID: 11135373]

[21]   Geng S, Zhou S, Glowacki J. Effects of 25-hydroxyvitamin D3 on proliferation and osteoblast differentiation of human marrow stromal cells require CYP27B1/1α-hydroxylase. J Bone Miner Res 2011; 26(5): 1145-53.
[http://dx.doi.org/10.1002/jbmr.298] [PMID: 21542014]

[22]   Woeckel VJ, Alves RDAM, Swagemakers SMA, *et al.* 1α,25-(OH)$_2$D$_3$ acts in the early phase of osteoblast differentiation to enhance mineralization *via* accelerated production of mature matrix vesicles. J Cell Physiol 2010; 225(2): 593-600.
[http://dx.doi.org/10.1002/jcp.22244] [PMID: 20506116]

[23]   Fomby P, Cherlin AJ, Hadjizadeh A, *et al.* Stem cells and cell therapies in lung biology and diseases: Conference report. Ann Am Thorac Soc 2010; 12: 181-204.

[24]   Chen YC, Ninomiya T, Hosoya A, Hiraga T, Miyazawa H, Nakamura H. 1α,25-Dihydroxyvitamin D3 inhibits osteoblastic differentiation of mouse periodontal fibroblasts. Arch Oral Biol 2012; 57(5): 453-9.
[http://dx.doi.org/10.1016/j.archoralbio.2011.10.005] [PMID: 22041016]

[25]   Chen K, Aenlle KK, Curtis KM, Roos BA, Howard GA. Hepatocyte growth factor (HGF) and 1,25-dihydroxyvitamin D together stimulate human bone marrow-derived stem cells toward the osteogenic phenotype by HGF-induced up-regulation of VDR. Bone 2012; 51(1): 69-77.
[http://dx.doi.org/10.1016/j.bone.2012.04.002] [PMID: 22521434]

[26]   Yamaguchi M, Weitzmann MN. High dose 1,25(OH)$_2$D$_3$ inhibits osteoblast mineralization *in vitro*. Int J Mol Med 2012; 29(5): 934-8.
[PMID: 22307202]

[27]   Jo S, Yoon S, Lee SY, *et al.* DKK1 Induced by 1,25D3 is required for the mineralization of osteoblasts. Cells 2020; 9(1): 236.

[http://dx.doi.org/10.3390/cells9010236] [PMID: 31963554]

[28]   Yamamoto Y, Yoshizawa T, Fukuda T, *et al.* Vitamin D receptor in osteoblasts is a negative regulator of bone mass control. Endocrinology 2013; 154(3): 1008-20.
[http://dx.doi.org/10.1210/en.2012-1542] [PMID: 23389957]

[29]   de Freitas PHL, Hasegawa T, Takeda S, *et al.* Eldecalcitol, a second-generation vitamin D analog, drives bone minimodeling and reduces osteoclastic number in trabecular bone of ovariectomized rats. Bone 2011; 49(3): 335-42.
[http://dx.doi.org/10.1016/j.bone.2011.05.022] [PMID: 21664310]

[30]   Kogawa M, Findlay DM, Anderson PH, *et al.* Osteoclastic metabolism of 25(OH)-vitamin D3: A potential mechanism for optimization of bone resorption. Endocrinology 2010; 151(10): 4613-25.
[http://dx.doi.org/10.1210/en.2010-0334] [PMID: 20739402]

[31]   Kogawa M, Anderson PH, Findlay DM, Morris HA, Atkins GJ. The metabolism of 25-(OH)vitamin D3 by osteoclasts and their precursors regulates the differentiation of osteoclasts. J Steroid Biochem Mol Biol 2010; 121(1-2): 277-80.
[http://dx.doi.org/10.1016/j.jsbmb.2010.03.048] [PMID: 20304055]

[32]   Takeda S, Yoshizawa T, Nagai Y, *et al.* Stimulation of osteoclast formation by 1,25-dihydroxyvitamin D requires its binding to vitamin D receptor (VDR) in osteoblastic cells: Studies using VDR knockout mice. Endocrinology 1999; 140(2): 1005-8.
[http://dx.doi.org/10.1210/endo.140.2.6673] [PMID: 9927335]

[33]   Nerenz RD, Martowicz ML, Pike JW. An enhancer 20 kilobases upstream of the human receptor activator of nuclear factor-kappaB ligand gene mediates dominant activation by 1,25-dihydroxyvitamin D3. Mol Endocrinol 2008; 22(5): 1044-56.
[http://dx.doi.org/10.1210/me.2007-0380] [PMID: 18202151]

[34]   Gu J, Tong XS, Chen GH, *et al.* Effects of $1\alpha,25$-$(OH)_2D_3$ on the formation and activity of osteoclasts in RAW264.7 cells. J Steroid Biochem Mol Biol 2015; 152: 25-33.
[http://dx.doi.org/10.1016/j.jsbmb.2015.04.003] [PMID: 25864627]

[35]   Feng X, Lv C, Wang F, Gan K, Zhang M, Tan W. Modulatory effect of 1,25-dihydroxyvitamin D3 on IL1 β -induced RANKL, OPG, TNF α, and IL-6 expression in human rheumatoid synoviocyte MH7A. Clin Dev Immunol 2013.

[36]   Rossini M, Maddali Bongi S, La Montagna G, *et al.* Vitamin D deficiency in rheumatoid arthritis: Prevalence, determinants and associations with disease activity and disability. Arthritis Res Ther 2010; 12(6): R216.
[http://dx.doi.org/10.1186/ar3195] [PMID: 21114806]

[37]   Kikuta J, Kawamura S, Okiji F, *et al.* Sphingosine-1-phosphate-mediated osteoclast precursor monocyte migration is a critical point of control in antibone-resorptive action of active vitamin D. Proc Natl Acad Sci 2013; 110(17): 7009-13.
[http://dx.doi.org/10.1073/pnas.1218799110] [PMID: 23569273]

[38]   Santos A, Bakker AD, Willems HME, Bravenboer N, Bronckers ALJJ, Klein-Nulend J. Mechanical loading stimulates BMP7, but not BMP2, production by osteocytes. Calcif Tissue Int 2011; 89(4): 318-26.
[http://dx.doi.org/10.1007/s00223-011-9521-1] [PMID: 21842277]

[39]   Saji F, Shigematsu T, Sakaguchi T, *et al.* Fibroblast growth factor 23 production in bone is directly regulated by $1\alpha,25$-dihydroxyvitamin D, but not PTH. Am J Physiol Renal Physiol 2010; 299(5): F1212-7.
[http://dx.doi.org/10.1152/ajprenal.00169.2010]

[40]   Zhao S, Kato Y, Zhang Y, Harris S, Ahuja SS, Bonewald LF. MLO-Y4 osteocyte-like cells support osteoclast formation and activation. J Bone Miner Res 2002; 17(11): 2068-79.
[http://dx.doi.org/10.1359/jbmr.2002.17.11.2068] [PMID: 12412815]

[41]   Lieben L, Masuyama R, Torrekens S, *et al*. Normocalcemia is maintained in mice under conditions of calcium malabsorption by vitamin D–induced inhibition of bone mineralization. J Clin Invest 2012; 122(5): 1803-15.
[http://dx.doi.org/10.1172/JCI45890] [PMID: 22523068]

[42]   Ito N, Findlay DM, Anderson PH, Bonewald LF, Atkins GJ. Extracellular phosphate modulates the effect of 1α,25-dihydroxy vitamin D3 (1,25D) on osteocyte like cells. J Steroid Biochem Mol Biol 2013; 136: 183-6.
[http://dx.doi.org/10.1016/j.jsbmb.2012.09.029] [PMID: 23064198]

[43]   St John HC, Bishop KA, Meyer MB, *et al*. The osteoblast to osteocyte transition: epigenetic changes and response to the vitamin D3 hormone. Mol Endocrinol 2014; 28(7): 1150-65.
[http://dx.doi.org/10.1210/me.2014-1091] [PMID: 24877565]

[44]   Arora J, Wang J, Weaver V, Zhang Y, Cantorna MT. Novel insight into the role of the vitamin D receptor in the development and function of the immune system. J Steroid Biochem Mol Biol 2022; 219: 106084.
[http://dx.doi.org/10.1016/j.jsbmb.2022.106084] [PMID: 35202799]

[45]   Athanassiou L, Mavragani CP, Koutsilieris M. The immunomodulatory properties of vitamin D. Mediterr J Rheumatol 2022; 33(1): 7-13.
[http://dx.doi.org/10.31138/mjr.33.1.7] [PMID: 35611096]

[46]   Shin D, Yuk J, Lee H, *et al*. A functional vitamin D receptor signalling. Nutrients 2010; 12: 1648-465.

[47]   Assa A, Vong L, Pinnell LJ, Avitzur N, Johnson-Henry KC, Sherman PM. Vitamin D deficiency promotes epithelial barrier dysfunction and intestinal inflammation. J Infect Dis 2014; 210(8): 1296-305.
[http://dx.doi.org/10.1093/infdis/jiu235] [PMID: 24755435]

[48]   Lin R. Crosstalk between Vitamin D Metabolism. VDR Signalling, and Innate Immunity 2016.

[49]   Zhang Y, Leung DYM, Richers BN, *et al*. Vitamin D inhibits monocyte/macrophage proinflammatory cytokine production by targeting MAPK phosphatase-1. J Immunol 2012; 188(5): 2127-35.
[http://dx.doi.org/10.4049/jimmunol.1102412] [PMID: 22301548]

[50]   Small AG, Harvey S, Kaur J, *et al*. Vitamin D upregulates the macrophage complement receptor immunoglobulin in innate immunity to microbial pathogens. Commun Biol 2021; 4(1): 401.
[http://dx.doi.org/10.1038/s42003-021-01943-3] [PMID: 33767430]

[51]   Jain SK, Micinski D. Vitamin D upregulates glutamate cysteine ligase and glutathione reductase, and GSH formation, and decreases ROS and MCP-1 and IL-8 secretion in high-glucose exposed U937 monocytes. Biochem Biophys Res Commun 2013; 437(1): 7-11.
[http://dx.doi.org/10.1016/j.bbrc.2013.06.004] [PMID: 23770363]

[52]   Hafkamp FMJ, Taanman-kueter EWM, Capel TMM, *et al*. Vitamin D3 priming of dendritic cells shifts human neutrophil-dependent Th17 cell development to regulatory T Cells. Front Immunol 2022; 13: 872665.
[http://dx.doi.org/10.3389/fimmu.2022.872665]

[53]   Kanikarla-Marie P, Jain SK. 1,25(OH)$_2$D$_3$ inhibits oxidative stress and monocyte adhesion by mediating the upregulation of GCLC and GSH in endothelial cells treated with acetoacetate (ketosis). J Steroid Biochem Mol Biol 2016; 159: 94-101.
[http://dx.doi.org/10.1016/j.jsbmb.2016.03.002] [PMID: 26949104]

[54]   Barragan M, Good M, Kolls J. Regulation of dendritic cell function by vitamin D. Nutrients 2015; 7(9): 8127-51.
[http://dx.doi.org/10.3390/nu7095383] [PMID: 26402698]

[55]   Bscheider M, Butcher EC. Vitamin D immunoregulation through dendritic cells. Immunology 2016; 148(3): 227-36.
[http://dx.doi.org/10.1111/imm.12610] [PMID: 27040466]

[56]   Carlberg C, Vitamin D. Vitamin D signaling in the context of innate immunity: Focus on human monocytes. Front Immunol 2019; 10: 2211.
[http://dx.doi.org/10.3389/fimmu.2019.02211] [PMID: 31572402]

[57]   Alvarez N, Gonzalez SM, Hernandez JC, Rugeles MT, Aguilar-Jimenez W. Calcitriol decreases HIV-1 transfer in vitro from monocyte-derived dendritic cells to CD4 + T cells, and downregulates the expression of DC-SIGN and SIGLEC-1. PLoS One 2022; 17(7): e0269932.
[http://dx.doi.org/10.1371/journal.pone.0269932] [PMID: 35802715]

[58]   Sonnenberg GF, Artis D. Innate lymphoid cells in the initiation, regulation and resolution of inflammation. Nat Med 2015; 21(7): 698-708.
[http://dx.doi.org/10.1038/nm.3892]

[59]   Rodríguez-Carrio J, Hähnlein JS, Ramwadhdoebe TH, *et al.* Brief Report: Altered innate lymphoid cell subsets in human lymph node biopsy specimens obtained during the at-risk and earliest phases of rheumatoid arthritis. Arthritis Rheumatol 2017; 69(1): 70-6.
[http://dx.doi.org/10.1002/art.39811] [PMID: 27428460]

[60]   Ferreira GB, Vanherwegen AS, Eelen G, *et al.* Vitamin D3 induces tolerance in human dendritic cells by activation of intracellular metabolic pathways. Cell Rep 2015; 10(5): 711-25.
[http://dx.doi.org/10.1016/j.celrep.2015.01.013] [PMID: 25660022]

[61]   Li C, Liu J, Pan J, *et al.* ILC1s and ILC3s exhibit inflammatory phenotype in periodontal ligament of periodontitis patients. Front Immunol 2021; 12: 708678.

[62]   Kindstedt E, Koskinen Holm C, Palmqvist P, *et al.* Innate lymphoid cells are present in gingivitis and periodontitis J Periodontol 2018; 17-0750.

[63]   Omata Y, Frech M, Lucas S, *et al.* Type 2 innate lymphoid cells inhibit the differentiation of osteoclasts and protect from ovariectomy-induced bone loss. Bone 2020; 136: 115335.
[http://dx.doi.org/10.1016/j.bone.2020.115335] [PMID: 32240850]

[64]   Ebbo M, Crinier A, Vély F, Vivier E. Innate lymphoid cells: Major players in inflammatory diseases. Nat Rev Immunol 2017; 17(11): 665-78.
[http://dx.doi.org/10.1038/nri.2017.86] [PMID: 28804130]

[65]   Momiuchi Y, Motomura Y, Suga E, *et al.* Group 2 innate lymphoid cells in bone marrow regulate osteoclastogenesis in a reciprocal manner via RANKL, GM-CSF and IL-13. Int Immunol 2021; 33(11): 573-85.
[http://dx.doi.org/10.1093/intimm/dxab062] [PMID: 34498703]

[66]   He L, Zhou M, He L, Zhou M, Li YC. Vitamin D / Vitamin D receptor signaling is required for normal development and function of group 3 innate lymphoid cells in the gut vitamin D / Vitamin D receptor signaling is required for normal development and function of group 3 innate lymphoid cells. ISCIENCE 2019; 17: 119-31.

[67]   Ruiter B, Patil SU, Shreffler WG, Diseases I, Hospital MG, Hospital MG. Diseases I, Hospital MG, Hospital MG. HHS Public Access 2016; 45: 1214-25.

[68]   Džopalić T, Božić-Nedeljković B, Jurišić V. The role of vitamin A and vitamin D in the modulation of the immune response with focus on innate lymphoid cells. Cent Eur J Immunol 2021; 46(2): 264-9.
[http://dx.doi.org/10.5114/ceji.2021.103540] [PMID: 34764797]

[69]   Konya V, Czarnewski P, Forkel M, Rao A, Kokkinou E. Vitamin D downregulates the IL-23 receptor pathway in human mucosal group 3 innate lymphoid cells. J Allergy Clin Immunol 2020; 141(1): 279-92.

[70]   Ercolano G, Moretti A, Falquet M, *et al.* Gliadin-reactive vitamin D-sensitive proinflammatory ILCPs are enriched in celiac patients. Cell Rep 2022; 39(11): 110956.
[http://dx.doi.org/10.1016/j.celrep.2022.110956] [PMID: 35705047]

[71]   Peelen E, Knippenberg S, Muris AH, *et al.* Effects of vitamin D on the peripheral adaptive immune

system: A review. Autoimmun Rev 2011; 10(12): 733-43.
[http://dx.doi.org/10.1016/j.autrev.2011.05.002] [PMID: 21621002]

[72]   Cantorna M, Snyder L, Lin YD, Yang L. Vitamin D and 1,25(OH)$_2$D regulation of T cells. Nutrients 2015; 7(4): 3011-21.
[http://dx.doi.org/10.3390/nu7043011] [PMID: 25912039]

[73]   Romao-veiga M, Rezeck P, Leticia M, Carlos J. Vitamin D modulates the transcription factors of T cell subsets to anti- inflammatory and regulatory profiles in preeclampsia. Int Immunopharmacol 2021; 101: 21-3.

[74]   Zaiss MM, Axmann R, Zwerina J, *et al.* Treg cells suppress osteoclast formation: A new link between the immune system and bone. Arthritis Rheum 2007; 56(12): 4104-12.
[http://dx.doi.org/10.1002/art.23138] [PMID: 18050211]

[75]   Kim YG, Lee CK, Nah SS, Mun SH, Yoo B, Moon HB. Human CD4+CD25+ regulatory T cells inhibit the differentiation of osteoclasts from peripheral blood mononuclear cells. Biochem Biophys Res Commun 2007; 357(4): 1046-52.
[http://dx.doi.org/10.1016/j.bbrc.2007.04.042] [PMID: 17462597]

[76]   Luo CY, Wang L, Sun C, Li DJ. Estrogen enhances the functions of CD4+CD25+Foxp3+ regulatory T cells that suppress osteoclast differentiation and bone resorption *in vitro.* Cell Mol Immunol 2011; 8(1): 50-8.
[http://dx.doi.org/10.1038/cmi.2010.54] [PMID: 21200384]

[77]   Levescot A, Chang MH, Schnell J, *et al.* IL-1β–driven osteoclastogenic Tregs accelerate bone erosion in arthritis. J Clin Invest 2021; 131(18): e141008.
[http://dx.doi.org/10.1172/JCI141008]

[78]   Kang SW, Kim SH, Lee N, *et al.* Response Elements in Its Conserved 2022.

[79]   Zhang X, Zhang X, Zhuang L, *et al.* Decreased regulatory T-cell frequency and interleukin-35 levels in patients with rheumatoid arthritis. Exp Ther Med 2018; 16(6): 5366-72.

[80]   Jeffery LE, Henley P, Filer A, Sansom DM, Hewison M, Raza K. Decreased sensitivity to 1,25-dihydroxyvitamin D3 in T cells from the rheumatoid joint. J Autoimmun 2018; 88: 50-60.

[81]   Hanggara DS, Iskandar A, Susianti H, *et al.* The role of vitamin D for modulating the T Helper 1 immune response after the coronavac vaccination. J Interf cytokine Res Off J Int Soc Interf Cytokine Res 2022; 42: 329-35.

[82]   Zhou Q, Qin S, Zhang J, *et al.* 1,25(OH)$_2$D$_3$ induces regulatory T cell differentiation by influencing the VDR/PLC-γ1/TGF-β1/pathway. Mol Immunol 2017; 91: 156-64.

[83]   Li B, Zhang X, Sun Z, *et al.* A novel strategy for the treatment of allergic rhinitis: Regulating Treg/Th17 and Th1/Th2 Balance *In Vivo* by Vitamin D. Comput Math Methods Med 2022; 2022: 1-7.
[http://dx.doi.org/10.1155/2022/9249627] [PMID: 35959353]

[84]   Saul L, Mair I, Ivens A, *et al.* 1,25-Dihydroxyvitamin D3 Restrains CD4+ T cell priming ability of CD11c+ dendritic cells by upregulating expression of CD31. Front Immunol 2019; 10: 600.

[85]   Shi Y, Liu Z, Cui X, Zhao Q, Liu T. Intestinal vitamin D receptor knockout protects from oxazolone-induced colitis. Cell Death Dis 2020.

[86]   Das M, Tomar N, Sreenivas V, Gupta N, Goswami R. Effect of vitamin D supplementation on cathelicidin, IFN-γ, IL-4 and Th1/Th2 transcription factors in young healthy females. Eur J Clin Nutr 2014; 68(3): 338-43.
[http://dx.doi.org/10.1038/ejcn.2013.268] [PMID: 24398649]

[87]   Wang F, Zhou L, Zhu D, Yang C. Retrospective analysis of the relationship between 25-OH-Vitamin D and diabetic foot ulcer. Diabetes Metab Syndr Obes 2022; 15: 1347-55.

[88]   Chen J, Bruce D, Cantorna MT. Vitamin D receptor expression controls proliferation of naïve CD8+ T cells and development of CD8 mediated gastrointestinal inflammation. BMC Immunol 2014; 15(1): 6.

[http://dx.doi.org/10.1186/1471-2172-15-6] [PMID: 24502291]

[89]   Ding Y, Liao W, He XJ, Xiang W. Effects of 1,25(OH)$_2$D$_3$ and vitamin D receptor on peripheral CD4 $^+$ /CD8 $^+$ double-positive T lymphocytes in a mouse model of systemic lupus erythematosus. J Cell Mol Med 2017; 21(5): 975-85.
        [http://dx.doi.org/10.1111/jcmm.13037] [PMID: 28063200]

[90]   Lysandropoulos AP, Jaquiéry E, Jilek S, Pantaleo G, Schluep M, Du Pasquier RA. Vitamin D has a direct immunomodulatory effect on CD8+ T cells of patients with early multiple sclerosis and healthy control subjects. J Neuroimmunol 2011; 233(1-2): 240-4.
        [http://dx.doi.org/10.1016/j.jneuroim.2010.11.008] [PMID: 21186064]

[91]   Yuzefpolskiy Y, Baumann FM, Penny LA, Studzinski GP, Kalia V. Vitamin D receptor signals regulate effector and memory CD8 T cell responses to infections. J Nutr 2014; 144(12): 2073-82.
        [http://dx.doi.org/10.3945/jn.114.202895]

[92]   Karkeni E, Morin SO, Tayeh BB, Goubard A, Nunès JA. Vitamin D controls tumor growth and CD8+ T cell infiltration in breast cancer. Front Immunol 2019; 10: 1307.

[93]   Bikle DD. Vitamin D and immune function: Understanding common pathways. Curr Osteoporos Rep 2009; 7(2): 58-63.
        [http://dx.doi.org/10.1007/s11914-009-0011-6] [PMID: 19631030]

[94]   Martens PJ, Gysemans C, Verstuyf A, Mathieu C. Vitamin d's effect on immune function. Nutrients 2020; 12(5): 1248.
        [http://dx.doi.org/10.3390/nu12051248] [PMID: 32353972]

[95]   Yamamoto EA, Nguyen JK, Liu J, *et al.* Low levels of vitamin D promote memory B cells in lupus. Nutrients 2020; 12(2): 291.
        [http://dx.doi.org/10.3390/nu12020291] [PMID: 31978964]

[96]   Shirakawa AK, Nagakubo D, Hieshima K, Nakayama T, Jin Z, Yoshie O. 1,25-dihydroxyvitamin D3 induces CCR10 expression in terminally differentiating human B cells. J Immunol 2008; 180(5): 2786-95.
        [http://dx.doi.org/10.4049/jimmunol.180.5.2786] [PMID: 18292499]

[97]   Sapra L, Bhardwaj A, Mishra PK, *et al.* Regulatory B Cells (Bregs) inhibit osteoclastogenesis and play a potential role in ameliorating ovariectomy-induced bone loss. Front Immunol 2021; 12: 691081.
        [http://dx.doi.org/10.3389/fimmu.2021.691081] [PMID: 34276682]

[98]   Tu KN, Lie JD, Wan CKV, *et al.* Osteoporosis: A review of treatment options. P&T 2018; 43(2): 92-104.
        [PMID: 29386866]

[99]   Weaver CM, Alexander DD, Boushey CJ, *et al.* Calcium plus vitamin D supplementation and risk of fractures: An updated meta-analysis from the National Osteoporosis Foundation. Osteoporos Int 2016; 27(1): 367-76.
        [http://dx.doi.org/10.1007/s00198-015-3386-5] [PMID: 26510847]

[100]   Reyes-Garcia R, Mendoza N, Palacios S, *et al.* Effects of daily intake of calcium and vitamin d-enriched milk in healthy postmenopausal women: A randomized, controlled, double-blind nutritional study. J Womens Health 2018; 27(5): 561-8.
        [http://dx.doi.org/10.1089/jwh.2017.6655] [PMID: 29676968]

[101]   Körmendi S, Vecsei B, Ambrus S, Orhan K, Dobó-Nagy C. Evaluation of the effect of vitamin D3 on mandibular condyles in an ovariectomized mouse model: A micro-CT study. BMC Oral Health 2021; 21(1): 627.
        [http://dx.doi.org/10.1186/s12903-021-01980-8] [PMID: 34876086]

[102]   Burt LA, Billington EO, Rose MS, Kremer R, Hanley DA, Boyd SK. Adverse Effects of High-Dose Vitamin D supplementation on volumetric bone density are greater in females than males. J Bone Miner Res 2020; 35(12): 2404-14.

[http://dx.doi.org/10.1002/jbmr.4152] [PMID: 32777104]

[103] Swart KMA, van Schoor NM, Lips P. Vitamin B12, folic acid, and bone. Curr Osteoporos Rep 2013; 11(3): 213-8.
[http://dx.doi.org/10.1007/s11914-013-0155-2] [PMID: 23873438]

[104] Zhang Y, Kou Y, Yang P, *et al.* ED-71 inhibited osteoclastogenesis by enhancing EphrinB2–EphB4 signaling between osteoclasts and osteoblasts in osteoporosis. Cell Signal 2022; 96: 110376.
[http://dx.doi.org/10.1016/j.cellsig.2022.110376] [PMID: 35690294]

[105] Dar HY, Azam Z, Anupam R, Mondal RK, Srivastava RK. Osteoimmunology: The Nexus between bone and immune system. Front Biosci 2018; 23: 464-92.

[106] Dar HY, Shukla P, Mishra PK, *et al.* Lactobacillus acidophilus inhibits bone loss and increases bone heterogeneity in osteoporotic mice *via* modulating Treg-Th17 cell balance. Bone Rep 2018; 8: 46-56.
[http://dx.doi.org/10.1016/j.bonr.2018.02.001]

[107] Dar HY, Pal S, Shukla P, *et al.* Bacillus clausii inhibits bone loss by skewing Treg-Th17 cell equilibrium in postmenopausal osteoporotic mice model. Nutrition 2018; 54: 118-28.
[http://dx.doi.org/10.1016/j.nut.2018.02.013] [PMID: 29793054]

[108] Sapra L, Dar HY, Bhardwaj A, *et al.* Lactobacillus rhamnosus attenuates bone loss and maintains bone health by skewing Treg-Th17 cell balance in Ovx mice. Sci Rep 2021; 11(1): 1807.
[http://dx.doi.org/10.1038/s41598-020-80536-2] [PMID: 33469043]

[109] Srivastava RK, Dar HY, Mishra PK. Immunoporosis: Immunology of osteoporosis—role of T cells. Front Immunol 2018; 9: 657.
[http://dx.doi.org/10.3389/fimmu.2018.00657] [PMID: 29675022]

[110] Sapra L, Azam Z, Rani L, *et al.* Immunoporosis: Immunology of osteoporosis. Proc Natl Acad Sci, India, Sect B Biol Sci 2021; 91(3): 511-9.
[http://dx.doi.org/10.1007/s40011-021-01238-x]

[111] Srivastava RK, Sapra L. The Rising Era of "Immunoporosis": Role of immune system in the pathophysiology of osteoporosis. J Inflamm Res 2022; 15: 1667-98.
[http://dx.doi.org/10.2147/JIR.S351918] [PMID: 35282271]

[112] Lu Y, Liu S, Yang P, *et al.* Exendin-4 and eldecalcitol synergistically promote osteogenic differentiation of bone marrow mesenchymal stem cells through M2 macrophages polarization via PI3K/AKT pathway. Stem Cell Res Ther 2022; 13(1): 113.
[http://dx.doi.org/10.1186/s13287-022-02800-8] [PMID: 35313964]

[113] Blijdorp ICJ, Menegatti S, Mens LJJ, *et al.* Expansion of Interleukin-22– and granulocyte–macrophage colony-stimulating factor–expressing, but not interleukin-17a–expressing, group 3 innate lymphoid cells in the inflamed joints of patients with spondyloarthritis. Arthritis Rheumatol 2019; 71(3): 392-402.
[http://dx.doi.org/10.1002/art.40736] [PMID: 30260078]

[114] Inanir A, Özoran K, Tutkak H, Mermerci B. The effects of calcitriol therapy on serum interleukin-1, interleukin-6 and tumour necrosis factor-α concentrations in post-menopausal patients with osteoporosis. J Int Med Res 2004; 32(6): 570-82.
[http://dx.doi.org/10.1177/147323000403200602] [PMID: 15587751]

[115] Liu F, Wen K, Li G, *et al.* Dual functions of lactobacillus acidophilus NCFM as protection against rotavirus diarrhea. J Pediatr Gastroenterol Nutr 2014; 58(2): 169-76.
[http://dx.doi.org/10.1097/MPG.0000000000000197] [PMID: 24126832]

[116] Bullock J, Rizvi SAA, Saleh AM, *et al.* Rheumatoid arthritis: A brief overview of the treatment. Med Princ Pract 2018; 27(6): 501-7.
[http://dx.doi.org/10.1159/000493390] [PMID: 30173215]

[117] Chu Y, Xu S, Wang J, *et al.* Synergy of sarcopenia and vitamin D deficiency in vertebral osteoporotic fractures in rheumatoid arthritis. Clin Rheumatol 2022; 41(7): 1979-87.

[http://dx.doi.org/10.1007/s10067-022-06125-y] [PMID: 35253099]

[118] Cai B, Zhou M, Xiao Q, Zou H, Zhu X. L-shaped association between serum 25-hydroxyvitamin D and all-cause mortality of individuals with rheumatoid arthritis. Rheumatology 2022.

[119] Mouterde G, Gamon E, Rincheval N, *et al.* Association Between Vitamin D deficiency and disease activity, disability, and radiographic progression in early rheumatoid arthritis: The ESPOIR Cohort. J Rheumatol 2020; 47(11): 1624-8.
[http://dx.doi.org/10.3899/jrheum.190795] [PMID: 31839594]

[120] Takaki-Kuwahara A, Arinobu Y, Miyawaki K, *et al.* CCR6+ group 3 innate lymphoid cells accumulate in inflamed joints in rheumatoid arthritis and produce Th17 cytokines. Arthritis Res Ther 2019; 21(1): 198.
[http://dx.doi.org/10.1186/s13075-019-1984-x] [PMID: 31470891]

[121] Sukharani N, Dev K, Rahul FNU, *et al.* Association between rheumatoid arthritis and serum vitamin D levels. Cureus 2021; 13(9): e18255.
[http://dx.doi.org/10.7759/cureus.18255] [PMID: 34712532]

[122] Mukherjee D, Lahiry S, Thakur S, Chakraborty D. Effect of 1,25 dihydroxy vitamin D3 supplementation on pain relief in early rheumatoid arthritis. J Family Med Prim Care 2019; 8(2): 517-22.
[http://dx.doi.org/10.4103/jfmpc.jfmpc_446_18] [PMID: 30984665]

[123] da Silva JLG, Passos DF, Bernardes VM, *et al.* Co-Nanoencapsulation of Vitamin D_3 and curcumin regulates inflammation and purine metabolism in a model of arthritis. Inflammation 2019; 42(5): 1595-610.
[http://dx.doi.org/10.1007/s10753-019-01021-1] [PMID: 31102126]

[124] Sakalyte R, Denkovskij J, Bernotiene E, *et al.* The expression of inflammasomes NLRP1 and NLRP3, toll-like receptors, and Vitamin D receptor in synovial fibroblasts from patients with different types of knee arthritis. Front Immunol 2022; 12: 767512.
[http://dx.doi.org/10.3389/fimmu.2021.767512] [PMID: 35126351]

[125] Myers LK, Winstead M, Kee JD, *et al.* 1,25-dihydroxyvitamin D3 and 20-hydroxyvitamin D3 Upregulate LAIR-1 and attenuate collagen induced arthritis. Int J Mol Sci 2021; 22(24): 13342.
[http://dx.doi.org/10.3390/ijms222413342] [PMID: 34948139]

[126] Vyas SP, Srivastava RN, Goswami R. Calcitriol attenuates TLR2/IL-33 signaling pathway to repress Th9 cell differentiation and potentially limits the pathophysiology of rheumatoid arthritis. Mol Cell Biochem 2021; 476(1): 369-84.
[http://dx.doi.org/10.1007/s11010-020-03914-4] [PMID: 32965596]

[127] El-Banna HS, Gado SE. Vitamin D: does it help Tregs in active rheumatoid arthritis patients. Expert Rev Clin Immunol 2020; 16(8): 847-53.
[http://dx.doi.org/10.1080/1744666X.2020.1805317] [PMID: 32783547]

[128] Kim H, Baek S, Hong S-M, *et al.* 1,25-dihydroxy Vitamin D3 and interleukin-6 blockade synergistically regulate rheumatoid arthritis by suppressing interleukin-17 production and osteoclastogenesis. J Korean Med Sci 2020; 35.

[129] Dankers W, González-Leal C, Davelaar N, *et al.* $1,25(OH)_2D_3$ and dexamethasone additively suppress synovial fibroblast activation by CCR6$^+$ T helper memory cells and enhance the effect of tumor necrosis factor alpha blockade. Arthritis Res Ther 2018; 20(1): 212.
[http://dx.doi.org/10.1186/s13075-018-1706-9] [PMID: 30236152]

[130] Zhou L, Wang J, Li J, *et al.* 1,25-Dihydroxyvitamin D3 ameliorates collagen-induced arthritis *via* suppression of Th17 Cells through mir-124 mediated inhibition of il-6 signaling. Front Immunol 2019; 10.

[131] Wen H, Luo J, Li X, Wei D, Liu Y. 1,25-Dihydroxyvitamin D_3 modulates T cell differentiation and impacts on the production of cytokines from Chinese Han patients with early rheumatoid arthritis.

Immunol Res 2019; 67(1): 48-57.
[http://dx.doi.org/10.1007/s12026-018-9033-4] [PMID: 30357602]

[132] Wen H, Liu Y, Li J, Wei D, Liu D, Zhao F. Inhibitory effect and mechanism of 1,25-dihydroxy vitamin D3 on RANKL expression in fibroblast-like synoviocytes and osteoclast-like cell formation induced by IL-22 in rheumatoid arthritis. Clin Exp Rheumatol 2018; 36(5): 798-805.
[PMID: 29465363]

[133] Primorac D, Molnar V, Rod E, *et al.* Knee Osteoarthritis: A review of pathogenesis and state-of-the-art non-operative therapeutic considerations. Genes 2020; 11(8): 854.
[http://dx.doi.org/10.3390/genes11080854] [PMID: 32722615]

[134] Woodell-May JE, Sommerfeld SD. Role of inflammation and the immune system in the progression of osteoarthritis. J Orthop Res 2020; 38(2): 253-7.
[http://dx.doi.org/10.1002/jor.24457] [PMID: 31469192]

[135] Askari A, Ariya M, Davoodi SH, Shahraki HR, Ehrampoosh E, Homayounfar R. Vitamin K and D status in patients with knee osteoarthritis: An analytical cross-sectional study. Mediterr J Rheumatol 2021; 32(4): 350-7.
[http://dx.doi.org/10.31138/mjr.32.4.350] [PMID: 35128328]

[136] Alabajos-Cea A, Herrero-Manley L, Suso-Martí L, *et al.* The Role of Vitamin D in early knee osteoarthritis and its relationship with their physical and psychological status. Nutrients 2021; 13(11): 4035.
[http://dx.doi.org/10.3390/nu13114035] [PMID: 34836290]

[137] Anari H, Enteshari-Moghaddam A, Abdolzadeh Y. Association between serum Vitamin D deficiency and Knee Osteoarthritis. Mediterr J Rheumatol 2019; 30(4): 216-9.
[http://dx.doi.org/10.31138/mjr.30.4.216] [PMID: 32467872]

[138] Montemor CN, Fernandes MTP, Marquez AS, Poli-Frederico RC, da Silva RA, Fernandes KBP. Vitamin D deficiency, functional status, and balance in older adults with osteoarthritis. World J Clin Cases 2021; 9(31): 9491-9.
[http://dx.doi.org/10.12998/wjcc.v9.i31.9491] [PMID: 34877283]

[139] Veronese N, La Tegola L, Mattera M, Maggi S, Guglielmi G, Vitamin D. Vitamin D intake and magnetic resonance parameters for knee osteoarthritis: Data from the osteoarthritis initiative. Calcif Tissue Int 2018; 103(5): 522-8.
[http://dx.doi.org/10.1007/s00223-018-0448-7] [PMID: 29943188]

[140] Rai V, Radwan MM, Agrawal DK. IL-33, IL-37, and Vitamin D interaction mediate immunomodulation of inflammation in degenerating cartilage. Antibodies 2021; 10(4): 41.
[http://dx.doi.org/10.3390/antib10040041] [PMID: 34842603]

[141] Amirkhizi F, Asoudeh F, Hamedi-Shahraki S, Asghari S. Vitamin D status is associated with inflammatory biomarkers and clinical symptoms in patients with knee osteoarthritis. Knee 2022; 36: 44-52.
[http://dx.doi.org/10.1016/j.knee.2021.12.006] [PMID: 35500429]

[142] Amini Kadijani A, Bagherifard A, Mohammadi F, Akbari A, Zandrahimi F, Mirzaei A. Association of serum vitamin D with serum cytokine profile in patients with knee osteoarthritis. Cartilage 2021; 13(1_suppl): 1610S-8S.
[http://dx.doi.org/10.1177/19476035211010309] [PMID: 33890506]

CHAPTER 5

Bone Water: Effects of Drugs on Bone Hydration Status

Mohammad Ahmed Khan[1,*]

[1] *Department of Pharmacology, School of Pharmaceutical Education and Research, Jamia Hamdard, New Delhi-110062, India*

Abstract: Water is the most crucial nutrient that constitutes roughly 20% of the cortical bone by volume, yet most ignored in health and nutrition areas. Hydration significantly influences the mechanical properties and tissue quality of bone, whereas bone dehydration causes an increase in its elastic modulus. Moreover, the low water content in the trabecular skeleton changes its construction (shrinkage) and leads to a significant alteration in mechanical properties. Numerous internal (a lack of thirst sensation) or external (polypharmacy or chronic consumption of certain drugs) factors cause hypohydration. Unfortunately, frail elderly individuals are more vulnerable to developing dehydration particularly, due to a decrease in the fat-free mass, which contains 73% of total body water. Today, technical advancements have led to an emerging understanding of how bone water changes in various conditions including aging, diabetes, osteoporosis, and osteogenesis imperfecta. Drugs may also change the impression of hypohydration through the increase of water elimination causing diarrhoea, diuresis, or sweat; a decrease in thirst sensation or appetite; or affecting the central thermoregulation mechanism. However, research on the interaction between bone hydration status and drugs/excipients has been insufficient. In the present review, we evaluate studies that focus on the significance of bone hydration and the effects of drugs/excipients on hydration status.

Keywords: Bone water, Total body water, Hypohydration, Bone mineral density.

INTRODUCTION

Age-related diseases are an inevitable feature of human biology, and the increasing prevalence of bone diseases is a reflection of society's age. The loss of bone mass is a consistent outcome of ageing both in men and women. However, loss of bone strength is far more critical than the loss of bone mass in determining the fracture risk [1]. Bone is a nanocomposite polymeric structure having primarily two components hydroxyapatite (mineral phase) and type 1 collagen

---

[*] **Corresponding author Mohammad Ahmed Khan:** Department of Pharmacology, School of Pharmaceutical Education and Research, Jamia Hamdard, New Delhi-110062, India; Tel: +91-9573206296; E-mail: khan.ahmed1511@gmail.com

Puneetpal Singh (Ed.)

(organic matrix) [2, 3]. The former provides strength and stiffness, whereas the latter influences the toughness of bone. The composite nature of bone cannot be completed without water which is 15-25% by volume, and almost 10% by weight (60% inorganic & 30% organic material), located in different sites, including loosely or tightly bound to the matrix or cortical part [4]. Water is equally significant for the mechanical and structural integrity of both cortical and cancellous bone [5]. Moreover, bone mineral density (BMD) and bone mass are strongly determined by the level of intracellular and extracellular bone water. The dependency of BMD and bone mineral content (BMC) on the level of total body water (TBW), extracellular water (ECW), and intracellular water (ICW) can be seen in transporting fluids in the bone tissue for proper nourishment. The narrow range of TBW is continuously renewed mainly by thirst and hormonal mechanisms and remains in the balance between intake and loss. Any disturbance in the mechanism will lead to dehydration. The dehydration of bone tissue leads to an increase in its hardness, and stiffness, and a decrease in energy and strain at fractures. Several factors such as ageing, sex, drugs, and diseases (diabetes and chronic kidney disease) can negatively impact the water content and lead to bone fragility and fracture. The chronic use of various medications can trigger dehydration or hypohydration by increasing water elimination through sweat, urination, or diarrhoea and also decrease thirst sensation, and altering thermoregulation [6]. Investigation of the bone water content has never been a mainstream subject of analysis. Its examination has been only conducted as a part of a more extensive quantitative analysis of other bone constituents. Therefore, our review will summarize the current understanding of bone water and how the alteration of body water can affect bone hydration and cause mechanical changes. Furthermore, we will evaluate the studies that have talked about the effects of drugs on the hydration status, and how bone water can be therapeutically modulated.

ROLE AND CONTENT OF WATER IN BONE

Bone is a highly heterogeneous composite tissue with every component of utmost importance in maintaining skeletal health. All the components have been studied extensively except water which is the least considered constituent even less than the endosteum, or osseous tissues. In mammalian bone, water comprises 20-25% of TBW. The water in bone exists in two states, bound or mobile/free/pore water. The water that exists in the extracellular space of intra-cortical pores including vascular space and lacuno-canalicular network is called free water. The lacunar-canalicular space contains osteocytes that are estimated at only 12% of the total volume of bone water and provide essential nutrients like glucose to the cells and transport solutes from the lacunar-canalicular system [7]. It means that water not only resides within lacunae, canaliculi, and vascular canals but is also found in other places like collagen matrix and mineral apatite/extracellular matrix [8]. The water found loosely or tightly bound to the matrix, and other mineralized tissues is called bound water [3]. Both kinds accomplish different roles and their interaction with other components is significant for the mechanical activity of the bone [9].The ratio of bound to free water describes the quality of bone tissue; it can be determined *in vivo* by imaging techniques such as magnetic resonance imaging (MRI). In cancellous bone, the water content is more than that reported in composed or cortical bone. The lower water content in cortical bone may be due to its higher density which can be correlated with its increased mineralization [10]. In a compact bone like femur, the difference in bone density and porosity varies along the length and circumference of the shaft. The porosity increases with age which lets the mobile water fill in pores and decreases the bound water content. It acts as a porosity marker in age-associated bone fragility [11].The water decreases with age due to increased mineralization. But, there is a conflict between studies; some suggest that the water content of cancellous bone decreases from birth to 30 years of age, and remains stagnant thereafter [12], while, another study has demonstrated a steadier loss of water content from birth to death [13]. In addition to that, various pathologies also cause alteration in bone hydration. In osteomalacia, the mineral content of the bone matrix decreases abnormally, and the water content increases correspondingly [12]. Similarly, a significant decrease in bone water has been found in women who had experienced an osteoporotic fracture [14]. Alteration in hydration due to ageing or disease can be a relevant marker in predicting bone diseases, fracture risk, and resistance. It could be better than a bone mineral density (BMD) evaluation. Water along with other components provides essential support like toughness, flexibility, and elasticity to the skeletal system. Hence, loss of water or dehydration affects the viscoelasticity of the tissue which increases tensile strength, stiffness, and hardness and decreases strain and energy to fracture of bone [15]. In ageing and osteoporosis, the amount of water decreases due to increased bone porosity. Thus, loss of toughness due to the less amount of water bound to collagen or increased collagen cross-links that displace water in the collagen matrix. It results in bone fragility [9]. Similarly, hydroxyapatite increases due to the mineralization of ageing bone till the age of 60 years which causes bone stiffness [16]. As the patient gets old, bones get stiffer due to increasing mineral content, and decreasing quantity of water resulting in brittle bone due to bone mineralization which is fracture-prone [16]. Another study has used solid-state NMR to elaborate on the role of water in bone and its association with bone constituents. Water forms structural support to the tissue by forming H-bonds support between the neighbouring ions [17]. The presence of crystal-bound water fills the vacancies and prevents the collapse of these crystallites. Furthermore, the water spread over the surface of mineral crystals helps in coupling the mineral phase with collagen phases, thus, serving to cushion protection against any mechanical stress. The water movement empowers the bone to face stress with minimal distortion. Another possible mechanism could be that under uniaxial tension, the water acts as a sacrificial layer to protect collagen from pruning [17].Water protects the bone from two major types of bone microdamage observed in humans, microcrack and diffuse damage [17]. Bone microdamage is caused by prolonged bone loading which accumulates microcracks in the cortical bone. However, bone hydration also plays a significant role in the occurrence and progression of microcracks [18, 19]. Bone loading cycles are greatly accumulated by the older bones such as Interstitial bone (part of cortical bone), therefore, the majority of microcracks occur in it. Higher levels of mineralization in the interstitial region result in decreased water content which potentially allows bone-cracking more easily [20]. Whereas, less mineralized bones are more prone to form diffuse damages [19]. However, very few studies have been performed on the role of water in the microdamage of bone. Moreover, some free water molecules get restructured during the load-bearing activity of bone, and vascular channels in bones provide passage to these free water molecules [21]. During loaded intervertebral compression, the disc loses water and continued loading for more than several hours leads to a decrease in disc hydration. Once the pressure on the vertebrae is relieved, the discs immediately reabsorb water and regain its volume. In this way, water performs signal detection to transfer information regarding the load-bearing environment. The intervertebral disc movements are also responsible for the influx of nutrients and the outflux of waste products [22, 23]. Ageing and osteoporosis significantly decrease the water content of the vertebral discs which leads to the loss of shock-absorbing capacity. Therefore, compression fractures are most frequent in old and osteoporotic patients [24]. The distribution of water with bone mineralization gives another insight into the vulnerability of bone to fracture in an elderly and postmenopausal population [9]. An early study has shown that decreased bone hydration has increased tensile stress, elasticity, and hardness of bone. It is possibly due to the water deficiency in the collagen fibres which makes them stiffer and stronger. However, the energy required for breaking a bone is higher for wet than dried bone [25]. The water found at the surface of bone mineral crystals may mechanically couple the mineral and collagen. Water plays a twofold function in the mammalian skeleton, one it provides a mineral reservoir for essential ions, and the other is that it offers a rigid weight supporter. It is a significant constituent of collagen in bone and tendons. The degree of hydration affects the mechanical properties of collagen [26]. The water attached to the collagen fibers delivers toughness to the bone, thus removing the water and increasing strength and stiffness (Fig. **1**).

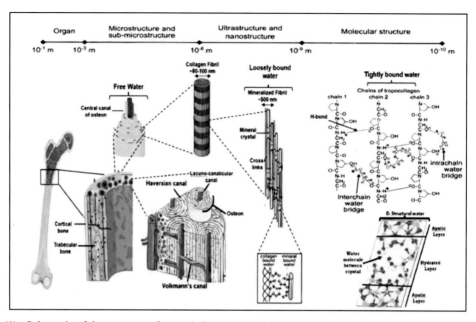

Fig. (1). Schematic of the presence of water in bone at each hierarchical level of organization.

LOCATION OF WATER IN BONE

Water is an important component, and its location decides the mechanical and structural integrity of bone. However, no studies have been done to recognize its location in the bone until 1969 when Blitz and Pellegrino identified and classified it as crystalline and osteoid [27]. Bone water can be free-flowing within pores, or it can be residing within a layer of mineral or collagen and can be called loosely, tightly and structurally bound water. Water molecules are located at different locations in the bone. In other words, bone water is found in four functional compartments, and each compartment contributes differently to the mechanical property of the bone. Some fraction of water exists in a free form called free water. Thus, it can freely move within vascular canals according to the pressure gradients that evolve during load-bearing skeleton movement. The free water molecule found in Haversian/Volkmann canals has a diameter of ~50-200 μm and ~0.1-5μm in lacunar-canalicular space [28]. It is also called pore water because of its occupancy within the macroscopic and microscopic pores of the tissue which likely participate in the hydraulic stiffness of the bone. Free water accounts for 20% of the total water present in bone [29]. Thus, an increase in free water content can lead to the loss of strength and gain of stiffness due to the inverse relationship between free water content and bone mass/mineral. However, increased free water content impairs cortical bone strength, mainly due to increased porosity rather than mineralization changes [30]. The relationship between free water and mineral implies that the more the amount of bone mineral, the less porous is the bone. Early studies used nuclear magnetic resonance (NMR) to determine free water and cortical bone porosity. Cortical bone porosity is defined as a major determinant of bone strength. It is responsible for the variation in the young modulus of the cortical bone up to 80% [31]. Ageing, hyperparathyroidism, osteoporosis (primary and secondary), and diabetes increase the porosity of the cortical bone [32 - 35]. Recognizing the role of bone porosity, various techniques have been introduced for *in vivo* assessment. Ultra-short echo time (UTE) and magnetic resonance imaging (MRI) allow for the evaluation of free bone water to determine porosity index values. It uses proton signals from free water present in bone pores, and bound water from collagen to correlate cortical porosity measured *via* micro-computed tomography (μCT) [36]. Free water found outside the pores helps in transmitting the signals from one cell to another through the streaming potential [37].

Around 20% of the wet weight of cortical bone is loosely bound water [38]. It is found between the collagen fibrils and mineral crystal layers and transfers load between them by sliding at their interfaces which helps in reducing the stress [39]. The binding energy required to bind the water molecule on the surface comes from the hydrophilic nature of the collagen molecules which draws the water into these mineral-collagen spaces [40]. However, current studies have found that glycosaminoglycans (GAGs) also have great affinity for both collagen and mineral crystals. Proteoglycans are non-collagenous containing GAGs and proteins found in the extracellular bone matrix. GAGs are negatively charged and highly polar, due to that reason it has a strong tendency to attract water molecules into the bone matrix *via* their osmotic gradient [41].

Loosely bound water resides within the organized surface of collagen and mineral crystals and can be physically adsorbed on the collagen or mineral surface to increase the gross toughness of the bone [42]. The rate of adsorption on the mineral surface declines with age and disease [11, 43]. It means the amount of loosely bound water and the toughness of bone decreases with ageing. During an experiment, loosely bound water was removed *via* drying, and the quality of young bone was affected more than elderly bone due to high porosity, less bound water, and low energy in the senile skeleton [43]. Similarly, removal of GAGs can lead to bone loss, bone toughness, and a decrease in biglycan (highly expressed proteoglycan in bone tissue) [7]. Quantification of loosely bound water with NMR methods is essential for the better assessment of fracture risk [44].

Some fraction of water (~0.5 gm) which is tightly bound with 1gm triple helix collagen is considered the backbone of collagen. More tightly bound water means greater toughness and lesser stiffness of the bone and vice versa [9]. It has been postulated that tightly bound water gives fibrillar structure to collagen because the removal of water from type 1 collagen shortens its length. It also ensures the efficient functioning of collagen at different temperatures [26]. Furthermore, there are water molecules that are incorporated around the mineral lattice and provide mechanical stability, which are called structural water. It forms the hydrogen bonding between ions in the mineral crystals. Thus, provides a medium for mineral plates to maintain organization and creates a continuous cross-fibrillar phase within unorganized collagen fibrils. Furthermore, it regulates the accumulation of minerals in the bone [45, 46].

VARIATION IN BONE WATER CONTENT

Whether free or bound, water plays a significant role in influencing the physical properties of the bone, and on the basis of water content, the tissue is differentiated into soft and hard. Reduced bone mass density is a conventional method to find out bone strength. However, it can only predict ~70% risk of fragility and fracture. Recent work has observed changes in bone water within the extracellular matrix due to ageing, pathology, and gender in the trabecular or cortex regions of bones [47].

Bone Type

Constituents like organic, inorganic and water make the essential components of the bone. The level of constituents increases or decreases according to the variety of bone. The low water content of the cortical bone can be correlated to increased mineralization [13]. Similarly, calcium is homogeneously distributed in the femur, whereas, no such uniform distribution can be found in flat bones. Therefore, the density of the femur is more than ribs and scapula [13]. Data obtained from *in vivo* study has revealed high water content in the scapula (12%) followed by ribs (11%), and femur (10%). Fractural change in bone density is the highest in the scapula and low in the ribs and femur. When these bones were oven-dried, the fractional change in density was the lowest in the femur than scapula or ribs [48]. However, if a bone is dried or decalcified, the variation in loss of density is significantly less.

Ageing

More than 50% of females and 25% of males face the incidence of fracture after the age of 50 years [49]. Ageing leads to sodium and water imbalances. Physicians face more than 11% of cases of acute hyponatremia in the elderly due to heavy loss of fluid which leads to a significant increase in plasma osmolality [50]. It further reduces the rate of bone blood flow which sharply enhances the risk of fracture in the elderly. Ageing causes bone porosity which increases the free water content in the extracellular matrix. In an aged skeleton, the number and size of pores positively correlate with the porosity index [36]. Recent studies have revealed that ageing leads to a progressive loss of bound water in bone, and collagen proteins, whereas mobile water doesn't decrease at the same rate [11]. These changes cause a 5-6% reduction in total water content in the ageing skeleton. According to a study, free water is negatively associated and bound water is positively associated with peak cortical bone stress. Whereas, bulk water does not have any association with the peak stress in aged bone [51]. Bound water is essential for the toughness and strength of bone which is eventually reduced up to 60% with age [51]. A femoral sample obtained from old mice has shown decreased bone toughness, strength, and bound water, but increased hyroxylysyl-pyridinoline and pentosidine crosslinking. Increased enzymatic and non-enzymatic cross-linking prevents the formation and removal of existing bound water in the aged skeleton. Increased amide-I sub-peak ratio also confirms diminished hydrogen bonding between mineral crystals and collagen residues, thus, decreasing bound water content [52, 53]. Aging-induced bone porosity causes bound water loss and higher glycation. It leads to bone loss in an ageing population. Therefore, direct measurement of pore water using imaging techniques can be used as a biomarker that can predict porosity.

Gender

Most studies on the skeletal system include male and female subjects, but there are significant differences between the bones of the two genders. According to various studies on postmenopausal osteoporosis, ageing, calcium or corticosteroids are not the primary causes of bone loss in females. The decreased production of estrogen is responsible for the change in the porosity of the bone.

Pathogenic Conditions

Osteoporosis is a metabolic bone disorder distinguished by reduced BMD (-2.5) and strength of the bone, and increased fracture risk [54]. In severe or persistent dehydration, the body requires an energy source, thus, it taps into the bones for their stored hydroelectric energy which could be the cause of bone fragility. Moreover, the porosity index also increases by 38% in an osteoporotic patient [36]. Pathogenic conditions like chronic kidney disease (CKD) also increase the risk of fracture. Various preclinical studies have mentioned higher levels of pore water in CKD rats. These animals have a high bone turnover number, as compared to the control group at 35 weeks [55]. However, in osteomalacia, the water content of the matrix is high as compared to the mineral content which softens the bone [12].

RELATIONSHIP BETWEEN BODY WATER AND BONE WATER

Water constitutes around 63% of the total body weight. Out of which, 73% is reserved in metabolically active fat-free mass (FFM) of the body (skeleton and skeletal muscle), whereas, fat reserves are practically devoid of water [56]. Previous studies on bone mass have confirmed a positive correlation between BMD and body water, and in a healthy adult, 60-70% of body mass is water along with calcium [57]. Water makes up to one-fourth of the total bone mass, and is a key component affecting the mechanical properties of bone. It is one of the important components that determine the BMD of bone [58]. Ageing shrinks down the FFM which could be the reason for decreased TBW, and bone mass in an elderly population. It reflects the dependency of bone tissues on TBW in obtaining minerals and body fluids for appropriate functioning and nourishment of bone tissue. Therefore, any changes in TBW can disturb the hemostasis of the body. TBW is further distributed in intracellular and extracellular compartments which ensure fluid balance and maintain the fluid shift in the body [59]. The distribution of water into different compartments also checks the fluctuation in hydration level. Loss of 12-15% of TBW can lead to death [57]. Tissues lacking water content are negatively correlated to the skeleton. Excessive fat reserves negatively affect bone health. Recent evidence finds that high body fat reduces body water which might not be beneficial for BMD [60]. It also influences inflammatory reactions that result in bone damage and can trigger inflammation-induced osteoporosis or immunoporosis [58]. Sarcopenic obesity reduces fat-free mass and increases the fat mass of the body, which is reported to be associated with bone loss in the elderly population [60]. In excessive obesity, relative increase in TBW and intracellular water might underrate the total body fat and overrate the fat-free mass [61]. Another study confirms a strong association between a water-less fat store with BMD. Increased body fat is significantly associated with a detrimental impact on the skeletal system [62]. The distribution of bone water in extracellular (ECW) and intracellular (ICW) compartments determines the BMD in the distal and proximal parts of the skeleton [57]. Most people do not associate body hydration with bone, but dehydration can lead to various bone pathologies. Drinking bicarbonate-rich mineral water has been found effective in improving BMD, bone microstructure, and biochemical properties in rats with metabolic acidosis [63]. Raloxifene, a selective estrogen receptor modulator (SERM) has an agonist effect on the skeleton, thus, being approved for the treatment of osteoporosis. Data has revealed that raloxifene decreases fracture risk by 50% and concurrently increases the TBW along with bone water after one year of treatment in postmenopausal females [64]. Furthermore, proteins present in the ECW like albumin maintain the colloid osmotic pressure in plasma, thus, playing a significant role in the distribution of fluid in the human body including bone [65].

CORRELATION BETWEEN DEHYDRATION AND BONE PATHOLOGIES

Water contributes to the bone's competency and affects both the mechanical and structural properties of bone. The interaction of water with bone components helps in maintaining microstructure (porosity and trabecular connectivity), macrostructure (curvature and cortical thickness), and micro- or diffuse cracks, thus, significant for the mechanical activity of bone [9]. During dehydration hardness, stiffness and tensile strength of the bone increase, and energy to fracture decreases (the ability of bone to resist fracture decreases). Similar observations have been noted in human dentine which loses plastic energy and toughness due to dehydration. However, these changes are reversible and abolished after rehydration [66]. There are several factors involved in bringing bone resorption, but one of the least considered is bone dehydration. A renowned physician Dr. Fereydoon Batmamgjelidj, gained international attention for his obstinate belief in water therapy and he described the possible relationship between osteoporosis and dehydration in his book. He said the gradual loss of thirst sensation or adipsia is the primary cause of chronic dehydration. The bone breakdown or osteolysis is brought about by prostaglandin E (PGE). The prolonged activation of PGE by histamine depletes calcium reserves of bone by osteolysis which exposes collagen for osteoclastogenesis. In this way, dehydration employs histamine to disbalance the rate of formation and resorption of bone [67, 68]. Furthermore, mast cell contains osmoreceptors that get activated during dehydration and release histamine [68]. The elevated mast cells probably promote osteoclast synthesis and also release other inflammatory osteoclastogenic mediators (TNF-α and IL-6). The treatment with calcium and promethazine helps in increasing BMD in postmenopausal women [69]. The dehydration mechanical properties of less mineralized bone-like trabeculae bear a greater impact as compared to more mineralized tissue like interstitial lamellae [70]. If a trabecular bone loses water, its behaviour becomes brittle, and its viscoelastic nature is also altered which hampers its recovery from strains [70]. Dehydration affects the properties of bone both at macroscopic and microscopic levels. A study found that dehydration removes the water from pores which impacts the viscoelasticity of cortical bone. It implies that the interaction of collagen, moisture, and minerals is significant for bone viscoelasticity [71]. The microindentation technique has been commonly used to identify the microhardness of bone. The diamond indenter is used to determine the hardness by pressing into the tissue with a known force. Indentation is an important technique to quantify the dehydration effect on mechanical properties of the skeleton. At the macroscopic level, dehydration increases the nanoindentation modulus of human vertebral and cortical bone [72, 73]. The tissue modulus of the cancellous bone increases by 28% due to drying. It contributes to the change in structure and material caused by dehydration [70].

Current studies have shown that the quality and mechanical resilience of bone lies in its microconstituents (water). Dehydration results in micro and macro changes in the structure and material of the bone which further increases tissue modulus by up to 27% and impacts the mechanical properties of bone [70].

DRUG-INDUCED WATER LOSS

The difference between water input and output is used to evaluate hydration status and determine the total fluid composition of the body. Thirst sensation, vasopressin secretion, renin-angiotensin-aldosterone system activation, sympathetic stimulation, and water excretion are several mechanisms that maintain hydration status in the body [74]. Water input is in equilibrium with water output but, that scenario is found during an ideal situation. During unwanted circumstances, water balance gets disturbed leading to dehydration or hypohydration. Undesired reasons could be anything that changes the hydration status including the use of medications. The influence of the drug on water level is not exclusive to the elderly, but the athlete and adult population could also be subjected [75]. The introduction of polypharmacy and chronic consumption due to certain drugs may also alter TBW. Generally, the drug affects the body's hydration through three mechanisms.

Drugs May Lead to Decreased Thirst

Increased plasma osmolality, decreased plasma volume, or decreased blood pressure are some of the thirst-stimulating factors [76]. Decreased thirst sensation is the most recognized characteristic of ageing, and it gets worse in case of any neurological disorder. Thirst perception is further depressed due to decreased function of the hypothalamus and pituitary glands [77, 78]. If the number of angiotensin 1 receptors decreases or osmoreceptors become irresponsive, it will aggravate the condition [78]. Along with the physiological changes, the use of multiple medications is another factor responsible for the decrease in thirst. An *in vivo* study has revealed that the renin-angiotensin system plays an important role in thirst perception, and inhibition of the system can cause a chronic reduction of thirst sensation. Chronic infusion of losartan significantly loses the sensation of thirst in mice. It reduces the water and salt intake thus leading to hypohydration [79]. An observational study has found that the use of renin-angiotensin aldosterone system (RAAS) inhibitors (ACE inhibitor and ARB's) for more than 3 years is associated with an increased risk of fractures in postmenopausal females [80]. Another study has found that the use of ACE inhibitors in females is associated with lower bone mineral density of the femoral neck and lumbar spine, and also lower trabecular bone score [81, 82]. Prolonged treatment of movement disorders (Parkinson's disease) with dopamine receptor agonists (D1 and D2) significantly reduces thirst sensation [83]. Similarly, antidepressants like venlafaxine, citalopram, clomipramine, duloxetine, clozapine, or risperidone are responsible for blocking thirst [84, 85]. An animal study on SSRIs has shown hyponatremia and inappropriate secretion of the anti-diuretic hormone (SIADH) thus reducing thirst sensation in rats [82, 86]. Interestingly, the chronic use of dopaminergic agonists is found to be associated with an increased risk of hip/femur fractures by multiple folds. Parkinson's disease patients also take antidepressants concomitantly which further increases the risk of fracture [87]. Another study has found that antidepressants reduce BMD and increase the risk of fracture. Similar effects have been found on the cell line, where antidepressant effects are seen on osteoclast and osteocyte cells. Thus, they hurt the skeletal system [88]. Despite having intriguing evidence, no human study has been designed to evaluate the association of thirst blockers with the onset of dehydration-associated fracture.

Drugs May Increase Water Elimination

Water is essential for existence, therefore, TBW is firmly maintained between ±0.2% of total body weight per day. The input and output of water from the body maintain the hydration balance. If the net loss of body water is around 1% of body weight, the plasma osmolality will increase, and if it goes beyond 2%, body performance will be impeded [89]. The ability of the body to maintain water balance can be affected by a change in physiology (ageing or illness) or drug use. Diminishing thirst sensation with aging makes the old population vulnerable to dehydration. It eventually decreases TBW along with the loss of FFM. Water elimination due to drugs is the most prominent reason for dehydration in the elderly [56]. Corticosteroids (CS) are potent anti-inflammatory and immuno-suppressive drugs that can induce diuresis in heart failure patients and animals [90, 91]. The explanation is given that CS increases the glomerular filtration rate due to its hemodynamic actions. Later, a study confirmed that CS-treated patients are more prone to suffer from dehydration [92]. Methylprednisolone treatment for 120 days lowered the strength of cortical and trabecular bone in male mice. The damage was greater than the treatment, the drug-related changes in bone microstructure, the value of bone hydration, and the non-conventional determinants of bone strength deteriorated by the 120th day. The CS treatment continuously decreased bone water and declined bone strength between days 60 to 120 [93]. Likewise, diuretics, theophylline, and empagliflozin increase urine formation. Diuretics have various side effects, and one of them is dehydration due to excessive urination. It causes the loss of essential electrolytes in susceptible older people. Diminishing thirst sensation makes it difficult to find out water loss until it's too late [94]. Continuous loss of body water due to ageing or use of drugs is associated with a loss of FFM hydration that may lead to a shift in body composition such as osteoporosis [95]. The incidences of most prevalent osteoporotic fractures (vertebral fractures) increase after the age of 55 years in females and 75 years in males. A large prospective study included females who found a high risk of vertebral and non-vertebral fractures in patients using diuretics. The positive relationship between thiazides and hyponatremia is expected to develop fractures independent of BMD and falls [96, 97]. Thiazide diuretics decrease free water clearance causing hyponatremia [50]. It reduces the potential of vertebrae to heal local microdamage which increases the risk of further fracture. Hyponatremia increases osteoclastic activity without increasing bone formation, thus, impairing bone repair and its quality without affecting BMD [28]. Current studies explain the relationship between thiazides and clinical vertebral fracture. A prospective study has reported increased vertebral fracture and loss of total hip BMD with loop diuretic use in older females [98]. In randomised controlled trials, one-year treatment with loop diuretic significantly decreased BMD and elevated bone turnover markers in subjects treated with bumetanide [99]. However, a possible mechanism behind that was different from thiazide diuretics. Loop diuretics increase calciuria which would decrease BMD [97]. Drug-induced alteration in plasma sodium reflects total body water status [50]. Oral antidiabetic, Gliflozin, or sodium-glucose cotransporter-2 (SGLT2) inhibitors are modern drugs that inhibit the reabsorption of glucose in the proximal tubules of the nephron and increase the excretion of glucose [6, 100]. The action is effective in lowering blood glucose levels without suppressing plasma insulin levels, but it leads to the loss of excessive water from the body. This increases the risk of dehydration [100]. Likewise, theophylline increases urine production, like diuretics by inhibiting solute reabsorption in the proximal nephron [101]. Some drugs decrease bone water with unknown mechanisms. In an osteoporotic ovariectomized rat model, alendronate (0.025 mg/kg/day) was used as a treatment drug. Later, a UTE MRI of the femur found decreased total water content. The decreased mean water content was paralleled with an increased mean degree of mineralization [102]. It explains the negative correlation between water and mechanical properties of bone.

FUTURE DIRECTION

From the available data, it can be concluded that very little is known about the role of water in bone. Although bone hydration is necessary for the mechanical and structural properties of bone, its removal from the extracellular bone matrix affects the mechanical property. This piece of knowledge has been obtained from imaging techniques, but many things are still unknown. The varied status of bone water with age, disease, and drugs, and its relation with TBW have allowed us to find more about its therapeutical significance. However, the role of drugs responsible for bone dehydration has not been researched so far. There are a large number of drugs that have a potential impact on HS, but few published studies answer this question. Therefore, careful review and prescription of a patient's medication are crucial for the prevention of drug-induced bone dehydration. Advancements in imaging techniques will enhance our ability to study hydration status in early diagnosis of bone diseases. Moreover, we need to know the ways to influence water distribution to enhance the fracture resistance ability of bone and develop novel therapies that can lower fracture risk.

CONCLUSION

Based on the available data, the role and relevance of water in bone are scarcely known in the arena of bone biology. Although hydration is necessary for the mechanical and structural properties of bone its depletion from the extracellular matrix affects the mechanical property. This piece of knowledge has been obtained from imaging techniques, but there are so many things that are still unknown. The varied status of bone water with age, disease, and drugs, and its relation with TBW have prompted scientists to find more about its therapeutical significance. However, the role of drugs responsible for bone dehydration has not been adequately examined so far. There are high numbers of drugs that have a potential impact on HS, but few published studies answer this question. Therefore, careful review and prescription of a patient's medication are crucial for the prevention of drug-induced bone dehydration. Advancements in imaging techniques will enhance our ability to study hydration status in the early diagnosis of bone diseases. Moreover, we need to know the ways to influence water distribution to enhance the fracture resistance ability of bone and develop novel therapies that can lower fracture risk.

REFERENCES

[1]   Hui SL, Slemenda CW, Johnston CC Jr. Age and bone mass as predictors of fracture in a prospective study. J Clin Invest 1988; 81(6): 1804-9.
[http://dx.doi.org/10.1172/JCI113523] [PMID: 3384952]

[2]   Broz JJ, Simske SJ, Greenberg AR. Material and compositional properties of selectively demineralized cortical bone. J Biomech 1995; 28(11): 1357-68.
[http://dx.doi.org/10.1016/0021-9290(94)00184-6] [PMID: 8522548]

[3]   Granke M, Does MD, Nyman JS. The role of water compartments in the material properties of cortical bone. Calcif Tissue Int 2015; 97(3): 292-307.
[http://dx.doi.org/10.1007/s00223-015-9977-5] [PMID: 25783011]

[4]   Boskey AL, Robey PG. The composition of bone.Primer on the Metabolic Bone Diseases and Disorders of Mineral Metabolism. Wiley Online Library 2018; pp. 84-92.

[5]   Ibrahim A, Magliulo N, Groben J, Padilla A, Akbik F, Abdel Hamid Z. Hardness, an important indicator of bone quality, and the role of collagen in bone hardness. J Funct Biomater 2020; 11(4): 85.
[http://dx.doi.org/10.3390/jfb11040085] [PMID: 33271801]

[6]   Puga A, Lopez-Oliva S, Trives C, Partearroyo T, Varela-Moreiras G. Effects of drugs and excipients on hydration status. Nutrients 2019; 11(3): 669.

[http://dx.doi.org/10.3390/nu11030669] [PMID: 30897748]

[7] Wang X, Hua R, Ahsan A, *et al.* Age-related deterioration of bone toughness is related to diminishing amount of matrix glycosaminoglycans (GAGs). JBMR Plus 2018; 2(3): 164-73.
[http://dx.doi.org/10.1002/jbm4.10030] [PMID: 30009278]

[8] Zhang D, Weinbaum S, Cowin SC. Estimates of the peak pressures in bone pore water. J Biomech Eng 1998; 120(6): 697-703.
[http://dx.doi.org/10.1115/1.2834881] [PMID: 10412451]

[9] Nyman JS, Roy A, Shen X, Acuna RL, Tyler JH, Wang X. The influence of water removal on the strength and toughness of cortical bone. J Biomech 2006; 39(5): 931-8.
[http://dx.doi.org/10.1016/j.jbiomech.2005.01.012] [PMID: 16488231]

[10] Miserez A, Schneberk T, Sun C, Zok FW, Waite JH. The transition from stiff to compliant materials in squid beaks. Science 2008; 319(5871): 1816-9.
[http://dx.doi.org/10.1126/science.1154117] [PMID: 18369144]

[11] Vaissier Welborn V. Environment-controlled water adsorption at hydroxyapatite/collagen interfaces. Phys Chem Chem Phys 2021; 23(25): 13789-96.
[http://dx.doi.org/10.1039/D1CP01028J] [PMID: 33942041]

[12] Mueller K, Trias A, Ray R. Bone density and composition: Age-related and pathological changes in water and mineral content. J Bone Joint Surg Am 1966; 48(1): 140-8.
[http://dx.doi.org/10.2106/00004623-196648010-00014]

[13] Timmins PA, Wall JC. Bone water. Calcif Tissue Res 1977; 23(1): 1-5.
[http://dx.doi.org/10.1007/BF02012759] [PMID: 890540]

[14] Vennin S, Desyatova A, Turner JA, *et al.* Intrinsic material property differences in bone tissue from patients suffering low-trauma osteoporotic fractures, compared to matched non-fracturing women. Bone 2017; 97: 233-42.
[http://dx.doi.org/10.1016/j.bone.2017.01.031] [PMID: 28132909]

[15] Sasaki N, Enyo A. Viscoelastic properties of bone as a function of water content. J Biomech 1995; 28(7): 809-15.
[http://dx.doi.org/10.1016/0021-9290(94)00130-V] [PMID: 7657679]

[16] Dey P. Bone Mineralisation.In Contemporary Topics about Phosphorus in Biology and Materials. IntechOpen 2020.
[http://dx.doi.org/10.5772/intechopen.92065]

[17] Wilson EE, Awonusi A, Morris MD, Kohn DH, Tecklenburg MMJ, Beck LW. Three structural roles for water in bone observed by solid-state NMR. Biophys J 2006; 90(10): 3722-31.
[http://dx.doi.org/10.1529/biophysj.105.070243] [PMID: 16500963]

[18] Boyce TM, Fyhrie DP, Glotkowski MC, Radin EL, Schaffler MB. Damage type and strain mode associations in human compact bone bending fatigue. J Orthop Res 1998; 16(3): 322-9.
[http://dx.doi.org/10.1002/jor.1100160308] [PMID: 9671927]

[19] Sahar ND, Hong SI, Kohn DH. Micro- and nano-structural analyses of damage in bone. Micron 2005; 36: 617-29.

[20] Sroga GE, Karim L, Colón W, Vashishth D. Biochemical characterization of major bone-matrix proteins using nanoscale-size bone samples and proteomics methodology. Mol Cell Proteomics 2011; 10(9): M110.006718.
[http://dx.doi.org/10.1074/mcp.M110.006718] [PMID: 21606484]

[21] Gun'ko VM, Turov VV, Shpilko AP, *et al.* Relationships between characteristics of interfacial water and human bone tissues. Colloids Surf B Biointerfaces 2006; 53(1): 29-36.
[http://dx.doi.org/10.1016/j.colsurfb.2006.07.016] [PMID: 16959475]

[22] Hall S. Basic biomechanics. 4th., McGraw-Hill Higher Education 2003.

[23]   Kraemer J, Kolditz D, Gowin R. Water and electrolyte content of human intervertebral discs under variable load. Spine 1985; 10(1): 69-71.
[http://dx.doi.org/10.1097/00007632-198501000-00011] [PMID: 3983704]

[24]   Ashton-Miller JA, Schultz AB. Biomechanics of the human spine and trunk. Exerc Sport Sci Rev 1988; 16: 169-204.
[http://dx.doi.org/10.1249/00003677-198800160-00008] [PMID: 2968912]

[25]   Max-Planck-Gesellschaft.Collagen: Powerful workout with water. 2015. Available from: https://www.mpg.de/8887201/collagen-tendons-bones

[26]   Masic A, Bertinetti L, Schuetz R, *et al.* Osmotic pressure induced tensile forces in tendon collagen. Nat Commun 2015; 6(1): 5942.
[http://dx.doi.org/10.1038/ncomms6942] [PMID: 25608644]

[27]   Biltz RM, Pellegrino ED. The chemical anatomy of bone. I. A comparative study of bone composition in sixteen vertebrates. J Bone Joint Surg Am 1969; 51(3): 456-66.
[http://dx.doi.org/10.2106/00004623-196951030-00003] [PMID: 4976035]

[28]   Seeman E, Delmas PD. Bone quality--the material and structural basis of bone strength and fragility. N Engl J Med 2006; 354(21): 2250-61.
[http://dx.doi.org/10.1056/NEJMra053077] [PMID: 16723616]

[29]   Biswas R, Bae W, Diaz E, *et al.* Ultrashort echo time (UTE) imaging with bi-component analysis: Bound and free water evaluation of bovine cortical bone subject to sequential drying. Bone 2012; 50(3): 749-55.
[http://dx.doi.org/10.1016/j.bone.2011.11.029] [PMID: 22178540]

[30]   Martin RB, Ishida J. The relative effects of collagen fiber orientation, porosity, density, and mineralization on bone strength. J Biomech 1989; 22(5): 419-26.
[http://dx.doi.org/10.1016/0021-9290(89)90202-9] [PMID: 2777816]

[31]   Currey JD. The effect of porosity and mineral content on the Young's modulus of elasticity of compact bone. J Biomech 1988; 21(2): 131-9.
[http://dx.doi.org/10.1016/0021-9290(88)90006-1] [PMID: 3350827]

[32]   Dickenson RP, Hutton WC, Stott JRR. The mechanical properties of bone in osteoporosis. J Bone Joint Surg Br 1981; 63-B: 233-8.

[33]   Kanis JA, Johansson H, Oden A, *et al.* A meta-analysis of prior corticosteroid use and fracture risk. J Bone Miner Res 2004; 19(6): 893-9.
[http://dx.doi.org/10.1359/JBMR.040134] [PMID: 15125788]

[34]   McCalden RW, McGeough JA, Barker MB, Court-Brown CM. Age-related changes in the tensile properties of cortical bone. The relative importance of changes in porosity, mineralization, and microstructure. J Bone Joint Surg Am 1993; 75(8): 1193-205.
[http://dx.doi.org/10.2106/00004623-199308000-00009] [PMID: 8354678]

[35]   Vu TDT, Wang XF, Wang Q, *et al.* New insights into the effects of primary hyperparathyroidism on the cortical and trabecular compartments of bone. Bone 2013; 55(1): 57-63.
[http://dx.doi.org/10.1016/j.bone.2013.03.009] [PMID: 23541782]

[36]   Rajapakse CS, Bashoor-Zadeh M, Li C, Sun W, Wright AC, Wehrli FW. Volumetric cortical bone porosity assessment with MR imaging: Validation and clinical feasibility. Radiology 2015; 276(2): 526-35.
[http://dx.doi.org/10.1148/radiol.15141850] [PMID: 26203710]

[37]   Liu J, Hou Z, Qin QH, Fu D, Pan S. Variation of streaming potentials with time under steady fluid pressure in bone. Appl Sci 2019; 9(18): 3726.
[http://dx.doi.org/10.3390/app9183726]

[38]   Ong HH, Wright AC, Wehrli FW. Deuterium nuclear magnetic resonance unambiguously quantifies

pore and collagen-bound water in cortical bone. J Bone Miner Res 2012; 27(12): 2573-81.
[http://dx.doi.org/10.1002/jbmr.1709] [PMID: 22807107]

[39]   Wang FC, Zhao YP. Slip boundary conditions based on molecular kinetic theory: The critical shear stress and the energy dissipation at the liquid–solid interface. Soft Matter 2011; 7(18): 8628-34.
[http://dx.doi.org/10.1039/c1sm05543g]

[40]   Surowiec RK, Allen MR, Wallace JM. Bone hydration: How we can evaluate it, what can it tell us, and is it an effective therapeutic target? Bone Rep 2022; 16: 101161.
[http://dx.doi.org/10.1016/j.bonr.2021.101161] [PMID: 35005101]

[41]   Wang X, Xu H, Huang Y, Gu S, Jiang JX. Coupling effect of water and proteoglycans on the *in situ* toughness of bone. J Bone Miner Res 2016; 31(5): 1026-9.
[http://dx.doi.org/10.1002/jbmr.2774] [PMID: 26709950]

[42]   Lees S. A mixed packing model for bone collagen. Calcif Tissue Int 1981; 33(1): 591-602.
[http://dx.doi.org/10.1007/BF02409497] [PMID: 6799171]

[43]   Ivanchenko P, Delgado-López JM, Iafisco M, *et al.* On the surface effects of citrates on nano-apatites: Evidence of a decreased hydrophilicity. Sci Rep 2017; 7(1): 8901.
[http://dx.doi.org/10.1038/s41598-017-09376-x] [PMID: 28827557]

[44]   Nyman JS, Gorochow LE, Adam Horch R, *et al.* Partial removal of pore and loosely bound water by low-energy drying decreases cortical bone toughness in young and old donors. J Mech Behav Biomed Mater 2013; 22: 136-45.
[http://dx.doi.org/10.1016/j.jmbbm.2012.08.013] [PMID: 23631897]

[45]   Duer M, Veis A. Water brings order. Nat Mater 2013; 12(12): 1081-2.
[http://dx.doi.org/10.1038/nmat3822] [PMID: 24257130]

[46]   Von Euw S, Chan-Chang THC, Paquis C, *et al.* Organization of bone mineral: The role of mineral–water interactions. Geosciences 2018; 8(12): 466.
[http://dx.doi.org/10.3390/geosciences8120466]

[47]   Allen MR, Burr DB, AllenMatthew R. Bisphosphonate effects on bone turnover, microdamage, and mechanical properties: What we think we know and what we know that we don't know. Bone 2011; 49(1): 56-65.
[http://dx.doi.org/10.1016/j.bone.2010.10.159] [PMID: 20955825]

[48]   Mohiuddin S. Change in bone density as a function of water content. Wor J Med Sci 2013; 8: 473-5248.

[49]   Sheer RL, Barron RL, Sudharshan L, Pasquale MK. Validated prediction of imminent risk of fracture for older adults. Am J Manag Care 2020; 26(3): e91-7.
[http://dx.doi.org/10.37765/ajmc.2020.42641] [PMID: 32181621]

[50]   Sunderam SG, Mankikar GD. Hyponatraemia in the elderly. Age Ageing 1983; 12(1): 77-80.
[http://dx.doi.org/10.1093/ageing/12.1.77] [PMID: 6846095]

[51]   Horch RA, Gochberg DF, Nyman JS, Does MD. Non-invasive predictors of human cortical bone mechanical properties: T(2)-discriminated H NMR compared with high resolution X-ray. PLoS One 2011; 6(1): e16359.
[http://dx.doi.org/10.1371/journal.pone.0016359] [PMID: 21283693]

[52]   Creecy A, Uppuganti S, Girard MR, *et al.* The age-related decrease in material properties of BALB/c mouse long bones involves alterations to the extracellular matrix. Bone 2020; 130: 115126.
[http://dx.doi.org/10.1016/j.bone.2019.115126] [PMID: 31678497]

[53]   Kopp J, Bonnet M, Renou JP. Effect of collagen crosslinking on collagen-water interactions (a DSC investigation). Matrix 1990; 9(6): 443-50.
[http://dx.doi.org/10.1016/S0934-8832(11)80013-2] [PMID: 2635757]

[54]   Das S, Crockett JC. Osteoporosis : A current view of pharmacological prevention and treatment. Drug

Des Devel Ther 2013; 7: 435-48.
[PMID: 23807838]

[55]   Allen MR, Newman CL, Chen N, Granke M, Nyman JS, Moe SM. Changes in skeletal collagen cross-links and matrix hydration in high- and low-turnover chronic kidney disease. Osteoporos Int 2015; 26(3): 977-85.
[http://dx.doi.org/10.1007/s00198-014-2978-9] [PMID: 25466530]

[56]   Ferry M. Strategies for ensuring good hydration in the elderly. Nutr Rev 2005; 63(6 Pt 2): S22-9.
[http://dx.doi.org/10.1111/j.1753-4887.2005.tb00151.x] [PMID: 16028569]

[57]   Kopiczko A, Adamczyk JG, Gryko K, Popowczak M. Bone mineral density in elite masters athletes: The effect of body composition and long-term exercise. Eur Rev Aging Phys Act 2021; 18(1): 7.

[58]   Wang H, Peng H, Zhang L, Gao W, Ye J. Novel insight into the relationship between muscle-fat and bone in type 2 diabetes ranging from normal weight to obesity. Diabetes Metab Syndr Obes 2022; 15: 1473-84.
[http://dx.doi.org/10.2147/DMSO.S364112] [PMID: 35586203]

[59]   Shimamoto H, Komiya S. The turnover of body water as an indicator of health. J Physiol Anthropol Appl Human Sci 2000; 19(5): 207-12.
[http://dx.doi.org/10.2114/jpa.19.207] [PMID: 11155349]

[60]   Scott D, Chandrasekara SD, Laslett LL, Cicuttini F, Ebeling PR, Jones G. Associations of sarcopenic obesity and dynapenic obesity with bone mineral density and incident fractures over 5–10 years in community-dwelling older adults. Calcif Tissue Int 2016; 99(1): 30-42.
[http://dx.doi.org/10.1007/s00223-016-0123-9] [PMID: 26939775]

[61]   Coppini LZ, Waitzberg DL, Campos ACL. Limitations and validation of bioelectrical impedance analysis in morbidly obese patients. Curr Opin Clin Nutr Metab Care 2005; 8(3): 329-32.
[http://dx.doi.org/10.1097/01.mco.0000165013.54696.64] [PMID: 15809537]

[62]   Chen YY, Fang WH, Wang CC, *et al.* Body fat has stronger associations with bone mass density than body mass index in metabolically healthy obesity. PLoS One 2018; 13(11): e0206812.
[http://dx.doi.org/10.1371/journal.pone.0206812] [PMID: 30408060]

[63]   Tan Y, Xu A, Qiu Z, *et al.* Drinking natural mineral water maintains bone health in young rats with metabolic acidosis. Front Nutr 2022; 9: 813202.
[http://dx.doi.org/10.3389/fnut.2022.813202] [PMID: 35387196]

[64]   Jacobsen DE, Samson MM, Emmelot-Vonk MH, Verhaar HJJ. Raloxifene and body composition and muscle strength in postmenopausal women: A randomized, double-blind, placebo-controlled trial. Eur J Endocrinol 2010; 162(2): 371-6.
[http://dx.doi.org/10.1530/EJE-09-0619] [PMID: 19884264]

[65]   Nishikawa H, Yoh K, Enomoto H, *et al.* Extracellular water to total body water ratio in viral liver diseases: A study using bioimpedance analysis. Nutrients 2018; 10(8): 1072.
[http://dx.doi.org/10.3390/nu10081072] [PMID: 30103528]

[66]   Jameson MW, Hood JAA, Tidmarsh BG. The effects of dehydration and rehydration on some mechanical properties of human dentine. J Biomech 1993; 26(9): 1055-65.
[http://dx.doi.org/10.1016/S0021-9290(05)80005-3] [PMID: 8408088]

[67]   Abdulrahman S. Water for Health, for Healing, for Life: You're Not SickYou're Thirsty. Warner Books 2020.

[68]   Goldstein DJ, Halperin JA. Mast cell histamine and cell dehydration thirst. Nature 1977; 267(5608): 250-2.
[http://dx.doi.org/10.1038/267250a0] [PMID: 405619]

[69]   Saxena Y, Routh S, Mukhopadhaya A. Immunoporosis: Role of innate immune cells in osteoporosis. Front Immunol 2021; 12: 687037.
[http://dx.doi.org/10.3389/fimmu.2021.687037] [PMID: 34421899]

[70] Lievers WB, Poljsak AS, Waldman SD, Pilkey AK. Effects of dehydration-induced structural and material changes on the apparent modulus of cancellous bone. Med Eng Phys 2010; 32(8): 921-5.
[http://dx.doi.org/10.1016/j.medengphy.2010.06.001] [PMID: 20638319]

[71] Yamashita J, Li X, Furman BR, Rawls HR, Wang X, Agrawal CM. Collagen and bone viscoelasticity: A dynamic mechanical analysis. J Biomed Mater Res 2002; 63(1): 31-6.
[http://dx.doi.org/10.1002/jbm.10086] [PMID: 11787026]

[72] Hoffler CE, Guo XE, Zysset PK, Goldstein SA. An application of nanoindentation technique to measure bone tissue Lamellae properties. J Biomech Eng 2005; 127(7): 1046-53.
[http://dx.doi.org/10.1115/1.2073671] [PMID: 16502646]

[73] Wolfram U, Wilke HJ, Zysset PK. Rehydration of vertebral trabecular bone: Influences on its anisotropy, its stiffness and the indentation work with a view to age, gender and vertebral level. Bone 2010; 46(2): 348-54.
[http://dx.doi.org/10.1016/j.bone.2009.09.035] [PMID: 19818423]

[74] McKinley MJ, Johnson AK. The physiological regulation of thirst and fluid intake. Physiology 2004; 19(1): 1-6.
[http://dx.doi.org/10.1152/nips.01470.2003] [PMID: 14739394]

[75] Walter AN, Lenz TL. Hydration and medication use. Am J Lifestyle Med 2011; 5(4): 332-5.
[http://dx.doi.org/10.1177/1559827611401203]

[76] Naitoh M, Burrell LM. Thirst in elderly subjects. J Nutr Health Aging 1998; 2(3): 172-7.
[PMID: 10995062]

[77] Begg DP. Disturbances of thirst and fluid balance associated with aging. Physiol Behav 2017; 178: 28-34.
[http://dx.doi.org/10.1016/j.physbeh.2017.03.003] [PMID: 28267585]

[78] Denaro CP, Brown CR, Jacob P III, Benowitz NL. Effects of caffeine with repeated dosing. Eur J Clin Pharmacol 1991; 40(3): 273-8.
[http://dx.doi.org/10.1007/BF00315208] [PMID: 2060564]

[79] Sakai K, Agassandian K, Morimoto S, *et al.* Local production of angiotensin II in the subfornical organ causes elevated drinking. J Clin Invest 2007; 117(4): 1088-95.
[http://dx.doi.org/10.1172/JCI31242] [PMID: 17404622]

[80] Carbone LD, Vasan S, Prentice RL, *et al.* The renin-angiotensin aldosterone system and osteoporosis: findings from the Women's Health Initiative. Osteoporos Int 2019; 30(10): 2039-56.
[http://dx.doi.org/10.1007/s00198-019-05041-3] [PMID: 31209511]

[81] Holloway-Kew KL, Betson AG, Anderson KB, *et al.* Association between bone measures and use of angiotensin-converting enzyme inhibitors or angiotensin II receptor blockers. Arch Osteoporos 2021; 16(1): 137.
[http://dx.doi.org/10.1007/s11657-021-01004-6] [PMID: 34536130]

[82] Stöllberger C, Finsterer J. Did thirst-blockers like angiotensin-converting-enzyme inhibitors, sartans, serotonine-re-uptake-inhibitors, dopamine agonists/antagonists, or atypical neuroleptics contribute to the exorbitant number of fatalities during the French 2003 heat wave? Pharmacoepidemiol Drug Saf 2007; 16(11): 1252-3.
[http://dx.doi.org/10.1002/pds.1456] [PMID: 17960864]

[83] Mittleman G, Rosner AL, Schaub CL. Polydipsia and dopamine: Behavioral effects of dopamine D1 and D2 receptor agonists and antagonists. J Pharmacol Exp Ther 1994; 271(2): 638-50.
[PMID: 7965779]

[84] De Picker L, Van Den Eede F, Dumont G, Moorkens G, Sabbe BGC. Antidepressants and the risk of hyponatremia: A class-by-class review of literature. Psychosomatics 2014; 55(6): 536-47.
[http://dx.doi.org/10.1016/j.psym.2014.01.010] [PMID: 25262043]

[85] de Leon J, Verghese C, Stanilla JK, Lawrence T, Simpson GM. Treatment of polydipsia and hyponatremia in psychiatric patients. Can clozapine be a new option? Neuropsychopharmacology 1995; 12(2): 133-8.
[http://dx.doi.org/10.1016/0893-133X(94)00069-C] [PMID: 7779241]

[86] Roehr J, Woods A, Corbett R, Kongsamut S. Changes in paroxetine binding in the cerebral cortex of polydipsic rats. Eur J Pharmacol 1995; 278(1): 75-8.
[http://dx.doi.org/10.1016/0014-2999(95)00099-7] [PMID: 7664815]

[87] Arbouw MEL, Movig KLL, van Staa TP, Egberts ACG, Souverein PC, de Vries F. Dopaminergic drugs and the risk of hip or femur fracture: A population-based case–control study. Osteoporos Int 2011; 22(7): 2197-204.
[http://dx.doi.org/10.1007/s00198-010-1455-3] [PMID: 20967420]

[88] Sansone RA, Sansone LA. SSRIs: Bad to the bone? Innov Clin Neurosci 2012; 9(7-8): 42-7.
[PMID: 22984652]

[89] Baldwin KM, Brooks GA, Fahey TD, White TP. Exercise physiology: Human bioenergetics and its application. 3rd., Mountain 2000.

[90] Berger S, Bleich M, Schmid W, et al. Mineralocorticoid receptor knockout mice: Pathophysiology of Na + metabolism. Proc Natl Acad Sci 1998; 95(16): 9424-9.
[http://dx.doi.org/10.1073/pnas.95.16.9424] [PMID: 9689096]

[91] Hunter RW, Ivy JR, Bailey MA. Glucocorticoids and renal Na + transport: Implications for hypertension and salt sensitivity. J Physiol 2014; 592(8): 1731-44.
[http://dx.doi.org/10.1113/jphysiol.2013.267609] [PMID: 24535442]

[92] Puga AM, Partearroyo T, Varela-Moreiras G. Hydration status, drug interactions, and determinants in a Spanish elderly population: A pilot study. J Physiol Biochem 2018; 74(1): 139-51.
[http://dx.doi.org/10.1007/s13105-017-0585-x] [PMID: 28799126]

[93] Dubrovsky AM, Nyman JS, Uppuganti S, Chmiel KJ, Kimmel DB, Lane NE. Bone strength/bone mass discrepancy in glucocorticoid-treated adult mice. JBMR Plus 2020; 5(3): e10443.
[PMID: 33778319]

[94] Armstrong L, Costill DL, Fink WJ. Influence of diuretic-induced dehydration on competitive running performance. Med Sci Sports Exerc 1985; 17(4): 456-61.
[http://dx.doi.org/10.1249/00005768-198508000-00009] [PMID: 4033401]

[95] Bossingham MJ, Carnell NS, Campbell WW. Water balance, hydration status, and fat-free mass hydration in younger and older adults. Am J Clin Nutr 2005; 81(6): 1342-50.
[http://dx.doi.org/10.1093/ajcn/81.6.1342] [PMID: 15941885]

[96] Jamal SA, Arampatzis S, Harrison SL, et al. Hyponatremia and fractures: Findings from the MrOS study. J Bone Miner Res 2015; 30(6): 970-5.
[http://dx.doi.org/10.1002/jbmr.2383] [PMID: 25294595]

[97] Paik JM, Rosen HN, Gordon CM, Curhan GC. Diuretic use and risk of vertebral fracture in women. Am J Med 2016; 129(12): 1299-306.
[http://dx.doi.org/10.1016/j.amjmed.2016.07.013] [PMID: 27542612]

[98] Lim LS, Fink HA, Blackwell T, Taylor BC, Ensrud KE. Loop diuretic use and rates of hip bone loss and risk of falls and fractures in older women. J Am Geriatr Soc 2009; 57(5): 855-62.
[http://dx.doi.org/10.1111/j.1532-5415.2009.02195.x] [PMID: 19368583]

[99] Rejnmark L, Vestergaard P, Heickendorff L, Andreasen F, Mosekilde L. Loop diuretics increase bone turnover and decrease BMD in osteopenic postmenopausal women: Results from a randomized controlled study with bumetanide. J Bone Miner Res 2006; 21(1): 163-70.
[http://dx.doi.org/10.1359/JBMR.051003] [PMID: 16355285]

[100] Mordi NA, Mordi IR, Singh JS, et al. Renal and cardiovascular effects of sodium–glucose

cotransporter 2 (SGLT2) inhibition in combination with loop diuretics in diabetic patients with chronic heart failure (RECEDE-CHF): Protocol for a randomised controlled double-blind cross-over trial. BMJ Open 2017; 7(10): e018097.
[http://dx.doi.org/10.1136/bmjopen-2017-018097] [PMID: 29042392]

[101] Liberopoulos EN, Alexandridis GH, Christidis DS, Elisaf MS, Mena R, Robert S. SIADH and hyponatremia with theophylline. Ann Pharmacother 2002; 36(7-8): 1180-2.
[http://dx.doi.org/10.1345/aph.1A425] [PMID: 12086552]

[102] Anumula S, Wehrli SL, Magland J, Wright AC, Wehrli FW. Ultra-short echo-time MRI detects changes in bone mineralization and water content in OVX rat bone in response to alendronate treatment. Bone 2010; 46(5): 1391-9.
[http://dx.doi.org/10.1016/j.bone.2010.01.372] [PMID: 20096815]

CHAPTER 6

Dietary Patterns and Rheumatoid Arthritis

Mahdieh Abbasalizad Farhangi[1,*] and **Ali Hojati**[1]

¹ Department of Community Nutrition, Faculty of Nutrition, Tabriz University of Medical Sciences, Tabriz, East Azerbaijan Province, 5166/15731, Tabriz, Iran

Abstract: Rheumatoid arthritis (RA) is a systemic autoimmune inflammatory disease that impairs patients' capacity to engage in everyday activities and deteriorates their quality of life. The disease develops in genetically vulnerable individuals *via* an autoimmune inflammatory process triggered by environmental stimuli. Diet and nutrition are potential environmental variables influencing the start and progression of the disease. Traditionally, nutrition and disease research has examined the relationships between individual nutrients, foods, or dietary groupings and risk factors with health outcomes. By examining food consumption in terms of dietary patterns, it is possible to gain complete knowledge of the combined effects of nutrients and foods on chronic illnesses. The Mediterranean, DASH, and vegetarian diets are preventive dietary patterns, whereas the Western diet stimulates RA activity.

Keywords: Rheumatoid arthritis, Dietary pattern, Mediterranean diet, DASH diet, Vegetarian diet, Western diet, Inflammation, Disease activity, Joints, Nutrients.

INTRODUCTION

Rheumatoid arthritis (RA) is a systemic autoimmune inflammatory disease that affects joints predominantly, with an approximate worldwide prevalence of 1% [1]. It has particular symptoms characterized by persistent inflammation that originates in the synovial membrane and leads to joint cartilage damage. It can lead to painful joint swelling, bone degradation, and the beginning of major bodily function impairments at an early age. RA has a negative impact on a patient's ability to do normal daily activities and can impair quality of life. Also, it entails a high economic burden on people and societies [2].

The disease develops in genetically susceptible individuals through an autoimmune inflammatory process caused by environmental factors [3]. Environmental factors such as smoking, air pollution, dust, and infections play an

* **Corresponding author Mahdieh Abbasalizad Farhangi**: Department of Community Nutrition, Faculty of Nutrition, Tabriz University of Medical Sciences, Tabriz, East Azerbaijan Province, 5166/15731, Tabriz, Iran; Tel: +98-9146496411; E-mail: abbasalizad_m@yahoo.com

Puneetpal Singh (Ed.)

important role in the etiology of the disease. Diet and nutrients are possible environmental factors impacting the onset and development of disease [4]. Accordingly, dietary intervention is commonly used to manage and reduce the symptoms of RA through multiple mechanisms, such as reducing inflammation, increasing antioxidant levels, modifying lipid profiles, and possibly altering the gut microflora [5].

Traditionally, studies on nutrition and diseases have investigated the associations between specific nutrients, foods, or food groups with risk factors and health outcomes. However, this approach has some limitations; the most important is that nutrients or food groups are not though diet is particular to the Mediterranean basinonsumed in isolation. It must be noted that "we don't eat nutrients, we eat foods," and that, in reality, we consume foods in specific patterns [6, 7]. In response to these limitations, a more comprehensive understanding of the combined impacts of nutrients and foods on chronic diseases may be obtained by exploring food intake in terms of dietary patterns. It is more applicable for clinicians and patients to focus on dietary patterns rather than particular nutrients in order to make beneficial dietary modifications to manage their disease [2, 8]. Regarding an individual's entire diet, a healthy dietary pattern provides nutritional adequacy, minimizes the risk of chronic diet-related diseases, and improves overall health [9]. Accordingly, in this chapter, we explore major dietary patterns that affect RA symptoms and development.

MEDITERRANEAN DIET

The Mediterranean diet is a plant-based dietary pattern consumed by people of countries bordering the Mediterranean Sea, particularly in Greece, southern Italy, and southern Europe (Fig. **1**). It is recognized as one of the world's healthiest dietary patterns, particularly for its role in preventing chronic diseases.

The Mediterranean diet is characterized by the following:

1. Daily consumption of non-refined cereals and other products (such as whole wheat bread, pasta, and brown rice), fresh fruits, vegetables, nuts, legumes and low-fat dairy products and limit refined sugars.
2. Frequent consumption of olive oil as the primary source of fat.
3. Moderate consumption of fish, poultry, potatoes, eggs, and sweets (It is advised that fish and seafood be consumed at least twice a week).
4. Monthly consumption of red meat.
5. Moderate intake of alcohol, preferably red wine, with meals.
6. Regular physical activity.

Although diet is particular to the Mediterranean basin, its principles are easily adaptable to accommodate foods and recipes from different cultures across the world [10, 11]. The scientific and public interest in the Mediterranean diet as a healthy and recommended eating pattern for the prevention and treatment of various health issues, including cardiovascular diseases, diabetes, arthritis, cancer, and obstructive sleep apnea, has increased considerably in recent years [12, 13].

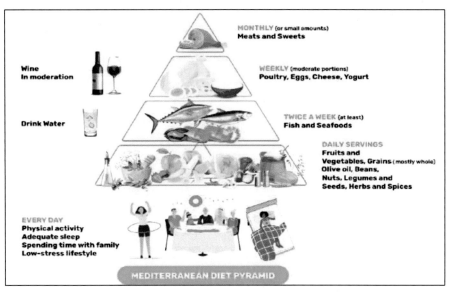

Fig. (1). The Mediterranean diet Pyramid.

However, there are contradictory studies regarding the effectiveness of the Mediterranean diet for RA. Sköldstam et al. found that the Mediterranean diet reduces disease activity in patients with stable and moderately active RA [14]. A significant reduction in disease activity score (DAS28) and overall health perception has been reported, as measured by the health assessment questionnaire (HAQ). Using the Short Form-36 (SF-36) questionnaire, increases in the individuals' quality of life were also seen. In another study, the intervention group showed significant improvements in terms of the disease's clinical characteristics, pain, morning stiffness, and health assessment perception after six months [15]. A population-based case-control study has demonstrated an inverse relationship between the Mediterranean diet and the risk of RA, but only in males with seropositive RA [16]. Another prospective study, investigated the association between adherence to the Mediterranean diet and the risk of getting RA in women in the United States [17]. The Mediterranean diet was evaluated using the Alternative Mediterranean Diet Index (aMed), which was calculated using the frequency of intake of nine food groups: whole grains, legumes, fruits, vegetables, fish, red meat, alcohol, and monounsaturated-saturated fatty acids. They reported that greater adherence to the Mediterranean diet might not provide major benefits for reducing the risk of RA since the components of this dietary pattern may have contradictory effects. In the Vasterbotten Intervention Program (VIP), a study reported that the Mediterranean diet was not correlated with the risk of developing RA [18]. To assess participants' adherence to the Mediterranean diet, they calculated the Mediterranean Diet Score (MDS) based on an FFQ of about 65 items.

Although controversial findings, adhering to the Mediterranean diet, which is rich in fish, olive oil, and vegetables, positively impacts the onset and development of RA. In considering the fact that inflammation might play a substantial and detrimental role in compromising health, it is evident that individuals who adopt the Mediterranean diet have reduced inflammation [19], including a decrease in proinflammatory biomarkers detectable in the systemic circulation, such as C-reactive protein (CRP), interleukin-6 (IL-6) and fibrinogen and better levels of oxidative stress indicators (*e.g.,* F2-isoprostane and total antioxidant capacity) [20].

Accordingly, the Mediterranean diet may help control inflammatory pathways in RA due to its high antioxidant and anti-inflammatory nutritional content [21]. This diet is an excellent source of polyphenols, rich in fruit, vegetables (especially herbs and spices), whole grains, nuts, seeds, and legumes. In addition, extra virgin olive oil and red wine (often excluded from other diets) include polyphenols (hydroxytyrosol, tyrosol, oleocanthal, and resveratrol), which are believed to have anti-inflammatory benefits. In addition, the Mediterranean diet contains small quantities of pro-inflammatory processed foods, beverages with high sugar content, and red meat [22]. Also, the long-chain omega-3 fatty acids found in fish and fish oil, which are precursors to anti-inflammatory eicosanoids, are believed to protect against the development of RA.

Prospective studies have demonstrated a negative association between dietary fiber consumption and inflammatory biomarkers such as IL-6, TNF-α, plasma fibrinogen, and hs-CRP [17].

Dietary fiber can also enhance gut microbiota composition and lowers joint discomfort in RA patients [23] (Fig. **2**). Therefore, eating nuts and whole grains may be effective in RA prevention. Furthermore, whole grains are abundant in anti-inflammatory antioxidants, such as vitamin E, phytic acid, and selenium, which may contribute to the anti-inflammatory process [17].

Consequently, the Mediterranean diet is a nutritionally sufficient, well-balanced diet that includes all food groups, and because it is not restrictive, it is more straightforward for patients to follow. However, there are few clinical studies, and more investigations are required to conclude its genuine effects.

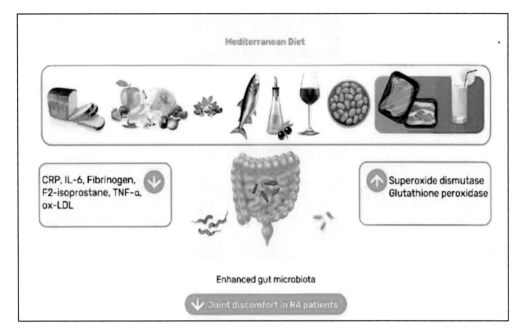

Fig. (2). Anti-inflammatory effect of Mediterranean diet on Rheumatoid Arthritis.

DASH DIET

Dietary Approach to Stop Hypertension (DASH) is an eating pattern that recommends higher consumption of whole grains, fruits and vegetables, low-fat dairy products, poultry and fish, and nuts and legumes. It also seeks to reduce the consumption of red meat, sweets, sugar-containing beverages, total fat, saturated fat, and cholesterol. Thus, the DASH diet encourages a higher consumption of essential nutrients such as potassium, calcium, magnesium, fiber, and vegetable proteins and a decreased consumption of refined carbs and saturated fat. The American Heart Association recommends DASH diet for the non-pharmacological treatment of hypertension. However, beneficial effects of the DASH diet are not limited to hypertension and blood pressure. It has been shown to enhance insulin sensitivity, inflammation, oxidative stress, and establish cardiovascular risk factors such as fasting glucose and total cholesterol levels [24].

Although studies investigating the direct association between DASH dietary pattern adherence and RA are limited, one study has indicated an inverse association between adherence to DASH dietary pattern and RA [25]. However, to overcome this limitation, it is essential to conduct more holistic studies to investigate the effect of DASH dietary pattern on RA rather than isolated nutrients.

The DASH diet includes plant-based foods high in antioxidants. Regular consumption may encourage a better balance between cellular oxidant and antioxidant systems and enhance the regulating of oxidizing (redox) processes in health and disease states [26]. Several studies have found that hs-CRP is correlated with disease activity. For instance, it is found that DAS28, a measure of disease activity in RA, is highly correlated with hs-CRP, and hs-CRP is correlated with disease activity [27]. It has been demonstrated that greater adherence to the DASH diet is related to decreased hs-CRP levels.

DASH diet is characterized by its high fiber, nut, and low-fat dairy content. Its high amounts of antioxidant minerals, including vitamins A, C, and E, are believed to be beneficial for their anti-inflammatory properties, which may lower CRP levels. In addition, this diet has a low glycemic index, which is negatively related to inflammation [28]. A meta-analysis has demonstrated that adherence to the DASH diet improves circulating serum inflammatory indicators in adults [29]. Hence, it may be a viable approach for suppressing the inflammation process.

VEGETARIAN DIET

A well-planned vegetarian diet can cover nutritional demands and be a healthy approach to fulfill dietary recommendations.

Typically, vegetarian diets fall into one of the following three categories:

1. Lacto-ovo-vegetarian is a diet modification that excludes all forms of animal protein other than dairy products and eggs. This diet is the most prevalent sort of vegetarian diet and the easiest to prepare.
2. Lacto-vegetarian is a diet modification that excludes all animal protein sources except dairy products. This necessitates making baked goods without eggs.
3. Strict vegetarian (vegan diet) is a dietary modification that excludes all forms of animal protein, also may exclude honey.

The more limited the diet, the harder it is to provide adequate nutrient intake. The vegan diet is more challenging but may be adequate with proper planning [30]. Formerly, vegetarian diets have been described as lacking in protein, iron, zinc, calcium, vitamin B12 and A, n-3 fatty acids, and iodine. Several studies have shown that deficits are typically the result of improper meal planning. Children, teenagers, pregnant and breastfeeding mothers, the elderly, and competitive athletes can all benefit from well-balanced vegetarian diets. Vegetarian diets are effective in preventing and treating various disorders, including cardiovascular disease, hypertension, diabetes, cancer, osteoporosis, renal disease, dementia, diverticular disease, gallstones, and RA [31].

In recent years, vegetarian diets for RA patients have attracted significant attention. A vegetarian diet high in fruits and vegetables and low in saturated fat may lower total body inflammation by modifying arachidonic acid, antioxidants, and essential fatty acids and decreasing food antigens [32].

In a randomized trial of patients with RA, the individuals completed a 7-10 days vegetable juice fast followed by a 3.5-month vegan diet. The patients were subsequently placed on a lacto-vegetarian diet for nine months. All clinical indicators, including sensitive and swollen joints, discomfort, length of morning stiffness, grip strength, and changes in an overall health evaluation, improved significantly in the diet group [33]. Further, a vegetarian diet can lead to reductions in concentrations of CRP, rheumatoid factor, DAS28 and Health Assessment Questionnaire (HAQ) scores [34].

Due to the high content of fruits and vegetables, the vegetarian diet can improve RA through anti-inflammatory and antioxidant properties. Additionally, a meta-analysis of twelve randomized controlled trials involving a total of 1151 subjects has shown that vegetarian diets, particularly vegan diets, appear to have significant beneficial effects on weight reduction [35].

Obesity is associated with increased disease activity as measured by the DAS28 in patients with RA, decreases the likelihood of disease remission in RA, and negatively affects disease activity and patient-reported outcomes throughout treatment [36]. Furthermore, the additional stress put on weight-bearing joints by excess weight worsens inflammation in these people; consequently, weight loss may be a beneficial treatment for RA [37] (Fig. **3**).

Also, gut microbiota and dietary fiber consumption may have a substantial effect on the activity of RA. A vegan diet decreases the relative number of Enterobacteriaceae in the gut, decreasing fecal lipocalin-2 (Lcn-2), a sensitive biomarker of intestinal inflammation, within 28 days [38].

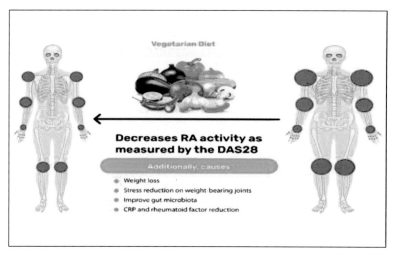

Fig. (3). Effect of Vegetarian Diet on DAS28.

WESTERN DIET

A 'Western' diet, in particular, with an increased intake of saturated and trans fats, a low ratio of omega-3: omega-6 fatty acids, an abundance of refined carbohydrates and sugar-sweetened beverages, and a low intake of fruits and vegetables, raises the risk of RA both directly and indirectly by raising insulin resistance, obesity, and related co-morbidities. Central to the Western dietary pattern, a high intake of red meat and meat products and total protein has been related to an elevated risk of inflammatory polyarthritis. Some possible mechanisms link the western diet to RA risk. Meat, fat and nitrites increase inflammation, and iron intake worsens inflammation in rheumatoid synovial membranes. Also, possible changes in gut microbiota and replacing the consumption of protective foods like fish with red meat are the possible mechanisms of the effect of the western diet on RA [39].

As formerly mentioned, obesity is associated with increased RA disease activity, and in recent decades, the western diet has significantly contributed to the increase in obesity rates. Western diet is associated with metabolic syndrome (MetS), and people with RA are also more likely to have MetS. A key aspect of MetS connected to RA is insulin resistance, which increases C-reactive protein, erythrocyte sedimentation rate, IL-6, TNF and disease activity ratings. On the other hand, beta-cell activity demonstrates an inverse relationship between DAS28 and a painful and swollen joint [40].

In addition to high amounts of unhealthy foods, the western diet is low in fruit and vegetables, making it an unhealthy dietary pattern that triggers RA activity (Fig. **4**).

OTHER DIETS AND RA

Studies of dietary patterns and dietary interventions on RA patients are limited. Effects of many dietary patterns have not been directly assessed in RA patients. Despite the evidence's limitations, we discuss other diets and food patterns that may positively affect RA directly or indirectly.

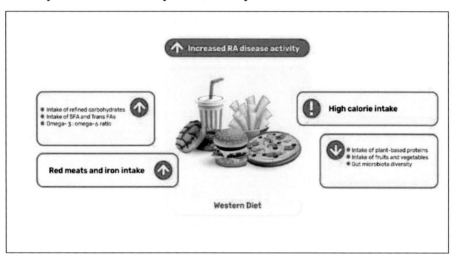

Fig. (4). Western diet can trigger RA activity.

Gluten-free Diet

Gluten, the primary storage protein of wheat grains, is a combination of two proteins called gliadin and glutenin, which are present in wheat, rye, and barley.

A gluten-free diet (GFD) is the only known effective treatment for celiac disease, an autoimmune condition characterized by an immunological sensitivity to gluten. GFD has also been studied as a potential therapy for different medical diseases, including dermatitis herpetiformis, irritable bowel syndrome, and RA [41]. A one-year gluten-free, vegan diet has been related to a substantial drop in anti-bet--lactoglobulin and anti-gliadin antibody levels and disease activity in RA patients [42]. Another study has shown that in patients with RA, a gluten-free vegan diet possibly causes atheroprotective and anti-inflammatory changes, such as lower LDL and oxLDL levels and improvements in DAS28 and HAQ scores [43]. In a case series study, patients with long-standing RA who were resistant to conventional and biotechnological drugs were treated by GFD simultaneously with drug therapy. Adherence to GFD led to a decrease in ESR, CRP, DAS28-CRP, and VAS. These results cannot be considered conclusive, but they can help partially explain the potential clinical outcomes of RA patients who commence a GFD [44].

It is important to note that no clinical trials have investigated the effect of a GFD without additional dietary modifications on disease outcomes in RA. Accordingly, in the absence of celiac disease, the French Society for Rheumatology's dietary recommendations states that a gluten-free diet should not be suggested to control the disease activity [45].

Intermittent Fasting

There are two primary types of intermittent fasting diets. Time-restricted feeding is the most prevalent form, which consists of a 16, 18, and 20-hour fast followed by an 8, 6, or 4-hour nutritional window. Reducing the nutritional window to four hours is a rigorous approach. Another strategy consists of alternating 24-hour periods of fasting and eating two or three times each week, with daily caloric intake during fasting periods ranging between 400 and 600 kcal [46]. A meta-analysis of 18 randomized controlled trials has reported that intermittent fasting, as compared to controls, has beneficial effects on inflammatory status, notably by lowering CRP levels [47]. In addition, based on treatment length and population type, a more considerable decrease in CRP levels has been found among overweight and obese individuals and for treatment durations lasting longer than eight weeks. According to one study, the treatment of RA is one of the most outstanding representatives of the favorable benefits of 1 to 3 weeks of long-term fasting, and RA patients experience a reduction in inflammation and joint discomfort while fasting [48]. However, when the usual diet is resumed, inflammation returns unless a vegetarian diet follows the fasting period. Therefore, fasting combined with a vegetarian diet and possibly other modified diets is effective for the treatment of RA. Also, alternate-day intermittent fasting leads to a substantial decrease in serum TNF-α in asthma patients. Moreover, indices of oxidative stress, frequently linked with inflammation, are considerably decreased in response to intermittent fasting. Another study has demonstrated that following the alternate-day intermittent fasting diet for four months lowers hs-CRP levels in individuals with MetS but has no effect on TNF-α and IL-6 levels [49]. Fasting has also been studied at the molecular level, resulting in lower IL-6 levels and disease activity. IL-6 has several functions in autoimmune diseases and can impact disease progression. However, in RA, its overproduction, notably in synovial cells and macrophages in the joints, corresponds to higher disease activity and joint destruction [50]. Furthermore, intermittent fasting helps people with chronic pain to feel less pain in the short term [51].

INDIVIDUAL FOOD ITEMS AND THEIR ROLE IN RA

Several studies have examined numerous dietary components and beverages regarding the risk of RA. Food items and nutritional factors can act as protective or trigger factors. Although the food items are not consumed in isolation, we cannot disregard the possible effects of different foods and nutrients on RA.

Dietary Fibers

Dietary fibers consist of soluble and insoluble components. The insoluble fibers have substantial bulking characteristics, while the soluble forms are fermented by particular gut microbiota species, resulting in active metabolites. Short-chain fatty acids (SCFA) are among the most numerous of these active metabolites, functioning as an energy source for intestinal epithelial cells, influencing the morphology and function of the gut, and providing energy for certain bacteria [52]. Dietary fiber can reduce local and systemic inflammation, and its modifying effects on gut bacteria diversity, SCFA synthesis, and intestinal barrier integrity can also reduce inflammation [37]. An inverse association has also been demonstrated between dietary fiber consumption and inflammatory biomarkers such as plasma fibrinogen, hs-CRP, TNF-α, and IL-6 levels, which are indicators of RA [53].

Fruits and Vegetables

Numerous health benefits are associated with the consumption of fruits and vegetables, which may be primarily attributable to their polyphenols and antioxidant characteristics. Fruits and vegetables can reduce RA risk [54, 55] and disease activity [56]. According to a study, ingestion of pomegranate extract for 8 weeks resulted in substantial decrease in DAS28, pain scores, HAQ, morning stiffness, and ESR as compared to individuals who did not consume pomegranate extract [57]. Berries and citrus fruits, among fruits, and green leafy vegetables, especially cruciferous vegetables, among vegetables, are to be preferred. Contrarily, tomatoes have been reported to worsen the symptoms of the disease [58].

Fish

Numerous studies have found an inverse relationship between fish consumption and the risk of RA. A study demonstrated that individuals who consumed fish 2 times per week or more had substantially lower DAS28-CRP levels than those who consumed fish <1 per month [59]. In another study each 30 g increase in daily consumption of high-fat fish (≥ 8 g fat/100 g fish) was related to a 49% reduction in the risk of RA. However, consuming medium-fat fish (3–7 g fat/100 g fish) was associated with a substantially increased risk of RA [60]. The role of fish in RA prevention is attributed to omega 3, an immune-modulating dietary component. Patients with RA who reported a larger consumption of omega 3 fatty acids and a lower omega 6 to omega 3 fatty acid ratio showed moderate or greater clinical improvement [61].

Olive Oil

The antioxidant effect of olive oil has been demonstrated to be beneficial for various health conditions, including cardiovascular disease and cancer. Consumption of olive oil also has been linked to a lower risk of RA [62]. Olive oil's beneficial effects on RA have been related to its fatty acid composition. It is rich in monounsaturated fatty acids (MUFA) and contains moderate amounts of saturated and polyunsaturated fatty acids (SFA and PUFA), as well as its high polyphenol and vitamin E content. All of these nutrients have anti-inflammatory properties and protect against immune-mediated inflammatory responses [58]. Moreover, a meta-analysis study has shown that olive oil consumption reduces some markers of inflammation (CRP and IL-6) [63].

Meat

Numerous studies have investigated the association between meat consumption and the risk of RA, but the results are limited and controversial. One study found that excessive red meat consumption raised the risk of inflammatory polyarthritis. However, it was uncertain whether the association was causative [64]. This association could be explained by increased inflammation caused by meat fatty acids and nitrites and increased synovial involvement caused by an excessive oral iron load [4]. However, several studies have shown no significant associations between meat consumption and risk of RA [60, 65 - 67]. Although association between red meat consumption and RA is unknown, it is important to underline that high meat consumption is usually a part of the Western Diet, which increases the risk of RA.

Dairy Products

Even though dairy products were formerly thought to be pro-inflammatory, research indicates that they have a neutral or anti-inflammatory effect on levels of circulating inflammatory biomarkers [58]. Dairy products have protective effects on RA and it has been reported that a lower intake of dairy products might relate to RA development [67]. Calcium is mainly consumed through dairy products. Patients with RA are more likely to develop osteoporosis due to the nature of their condition and their frequent and continuous exposure to corticosteroids. Accordingly, it is not recommended to eliminate dairy products for managing RA [45].

Salt

High sodium (salt) consumption, as seen in the Western diet, has been related to an increased risk of rheumatoid arthritis. There is evidence that increased salt intake activates proinflammatory macrophages (M1) and Th17 cells and decreases T-regulator cells (Treg), which have an essential role in the pathophysiology of RA. In addition, sodium excretion has been shown to be higher in early RA patients than in controls [4]. The evidence suggests that reducing salt intake might be beneficial in RA treatment.

CONCLUSION

Different studies indicate that diet has a critical role in managing RA by regulating inflammation, immunity, and oxidative stress. Although studies on dietary patterns and RA are limited and controversial, adherence to healthy dietary patterns (*e.g.,* Mediterranean diet, DASH diet, and vegetarian diet) can improve RA activity and decrease disease development. On the other hand, unhealthy diets, with characteristics similar to the Western diet, can worsen inflammation and RA status in patients. There are also some diets that may be hard to adhere to but can improve RA, like a Gluten-free diet and intermittent fasting. Furthermore, some individual food items may act as protective (*e.g.,* olive oil, dietary fiber) or trigger factors (*e.g.,* salt). However, it is essential to note that considering food intake in terms of dietary patterns makes it feasible to acquire a comprehensive understanding of the combined impact of nutrients and foods on chronic diseases.

REFERENCES

[1]   Smolen JS, Aletaha D, Barton A, *et al.* Rheumatoid arthritis. Nat Rev Dis Primers 2018; 4(1): 18001.
        [http://dx.doi.org/10.1038/nrdp.2018.1] [PMID: 29417936]

[2]   Nezamoleslami S, Ghiasvand R, Feizi A, Salesi M, Pourmasoumi M. The relationship between dietary patterns and rheumatoid arthritis: A case–control study. Nutr Metab 2020; 17(1): 75.
        [http://dx.doi.org/10.1186/s12986-020-00502-7] [PMID: 32963579]

[3]   Skoczyńska M, Świerkot J. The role of diet in rheumatoid arthritis. Reumatologia 2018; 56(4): 259-67.
        [http://dx.doi.org/10.5114/reum.2018.77979] [PMID: 30237632]

[4]   Gioia C, Lucchino B, Tarsitano MG, Iannuccelli C, Di Franco M. Dietary habits and nutrition in rheumatoid arthritis: Can diet influence disease development and clinical manifestations? Nutrients 2020; 12(5): 1456.
        [http://dx.doi.org/10.3390/nu12051456] [PMID: 32443535]

[5]   Forsyth C, Kouvari M, D'Cunha NM, *et al.* The effects of the mediterranean diet on rheumatoid arthritis prevention and treatment: A systematic review of human prospective studies. Rheumatol Int 2018; 38(5): 737-47.
        [http://dx.doi.org/10.1007/s00296-017-3912-1] [PMID: 29256100]

[6]   Calder PC, Ahluwalia N, Brouns F, *et al.* Dietary factors and low-grade inflammation in relation to overweight and obesity. Br J Nutr 2011; 106(S3) (3): S5-S78.
        [http://dx.doi.org/10.1017/S0007114511005460] [PMID: 22133051]

[7]   Mosalmanzadeh N, Jandari S, Soleimani D, *et al.* Major dietary patterns and food groups in relation to rheumatoid arthritis in newly diagnosed patients. Food Sci Nutr 2020; 8(12): 6477-86.
[http://dx.doi.org/10.1002/fsn3.1938] [PMID: 33312533]

[8]   Sparks JA, Barbhaiya M, Tedeschi SK, *et al.* Inflammatory dietary pattern and risk of developing rheumatoid arthritis in women. Clin Rheumatol 2019; 38(1): 243-50.
[http://dx.doi.org/10.1007/s10067-018-4261-5] [PMID: 30109509]

[9]   Okubo H, Sasaki S, Murakami K, Takahashi Y. Nutritional adequacy of four dietary patterns defined by cluster analysis in Japanese women aged 18-20 years. Asia Pac J Clin Nutr 2010; 19(4): 555-63.
[PMID: 21147718]

[10]   Donovan MG, Selmin OI, Doetschman TC, Romagnolo DF. Mediterranean diet: Prevention of colorectal cancer. Front Nutr 2017; 4: 59.
[http://dx.doi.org/10.3389/fnut.2017.00059] [PMID: 29259973]

[11]   Finicelli M, Di Salle A, Galderisi U, Peluso G. The mediterranean diet: An update of the clinical trials. Nutrients 2022; 14(14): 2956.
[http://dx.doi.org/10.3390/nu14142956] [PMID: 35889911]

[12]   Winkvist A, Bärebring L, Gjertsson I, Ellegård L, Lindqvist HM. A randomized controlled cross-over trial investigating the effect of anti-inflammatory diet on disease activity and quality of life in rheumatoid arthritis: The anti-inflammatory diet in rheumatoid arthritis (ADIRA) study protocol. Nutr J 2018; 17(1): 44.
[http://dx.doi.org/10.1186/s12937-018-0354-x] [PMID: 29678183]

[13]   Dobrosielski DA, Papandreou C, Patil SP, Salas-Salvadó J. Diet and exercise in the management of obstructive sleep apnoea and cardiovascular disease risk. Eur Respir Rev 2017; 26(144): 160110.
[http://dx.doi.org/10.1183/16000617.0110-2016] [PMID: 28659501]

[14]   Sköldstam L, Hagfors L, Johansson G. An experimental study of a Mediterranean diet intervention for patients with rheumatoid arthritis. Ann Rheum Dis 2003; 62(3): 208-14.
[http://dx.doi.org/10.1136/ard.62.3.208] [PMID: 12594104]

[15]   McKellar G, Morrison E, McEntegart A, *et al.* A pilot study of a Mediterranean-type diet intervention in female patients with rheumatoid arthritis living in areas of social deprivation in Glasgow. Ann Rheum Dis 2007; 66(9): 1239-43.
[http://dx.doi.org/10.1136/ard.2006.065151] [PMID: 17613557]

[16]   Johansson K, Askling J, Alfredsson L, Di Giuseppe D. Mediterranean diet and risk of rheumatoid arthritis: a population-based case-control study. Arthritis Res Ther 2018; 20(1): 175.
[http://dx.doi.org/10.1186/s13075-018-1680-2] [PMID: 30092814]

[17]   Hu Y, Costenbader Kh Fau, Gao X, *et al.* Mediterranean diet and incidence of rheumatoid arthritis in women. Electronic 2016; pp. 2151-4658.

[18]   Sundström B, Johansson I, Rantapää-Dahlqvist S. Diet and alcohol as risk factors for rheumatoid arthritis: A nested case–control study. Rheumatol Int 2015; 35(3): 533-9.
[http://dx.doi.org/10.1007/s00296-014-3185-x] [PMID: 25428595]

[19]   Tsigalou C, Konstantinidis T, Paraschaki A, Stavropoulou E, Voidarou C, Bezirtzoglou E. Mediterranean diet as a tool to combat inflammation and chronic diseases. an overview. Biomedicines 2020; 8(7): 201.
[http://dx.doi.org/10.3390/biomedicines8070201] [PMID: 32650619]

[20]   Aleksandrova K, Koelman L, Rodrigues CE. Dietary patterns and biomarkers of oxidative stress and inflammation: A systematic review of observational and intervention studies. Redox Biol 2021; 42: 101869.
[http://dx.doi.org/10.1016/j.redox.2021.101869] [PMID: 33541846]

[21]   Petersson S, Philippou E, Rodomar C, Nikiphorou E. The Mediterranean diet, fish oil supplements and Rheumatoid arthritis outcomes: Evidence from clinical trials. Autoimmun Rev 2018; 17(11): 1105-14.

[http://dx.doi.org/10.1016/j.autrev.2018.06.007] [PMID: 30213690]

[22]   Beam A, Clinger E, Hao L. Effect of diet and dietary components on the composition of the gut microbiota. Nutrients 2021; 13(8): 2795.
[http://dx.doi.org/10.3390/nu13082795] [PMID: 34444955]

[23]   Zhao T, Wei Y, Zhu Y, *et al.* Gut microbiota and rheumatoid arthritis: From pathogenesis to novel therapeutic opportunities. Front Immunol 2022; 13: 1007165.
[http://dx.doi.org/10.3389/fimmu.2022.1007165] [PMID: 36159786]

[24]   Siervo M, Lara J, Chowdhury S, Ashor A, Oggioni C, Mathers JC. Effects of the dietary approach to stop hypertension (dash) diet on cardiovascular risk factors: A systematic review and meta-analysis. Br J Nutr 2015; 113(1): 1-15.
[http://dx.doi.org/10.1017/S0007114514003341] [PMID: 25430608]

[25]   Ghaseminasabparizi M, Nazarinia MA, Akhlaghi M. Adherence to the dietary approaches to stop hypertension dietary pattern and rheumatoid arthritis in Iranian adults. Public Health Nutr 2021; 24(18): 6085-93.
[http://dx.doi.org/10.1017/S1368980021003608] [PMID: 34412722]

[26]   Mills CE, Khatri J, Maskell P, Odongerel C, Webb AJ. It is rocket science ; Why dietary nitrate is hard to 'beet'! *Part II : Further mechanisms and therapeutic potential of the nitrate-nitrite-NO pathway.* Br J Clin Pharmacol 2017; 83(1): 140-51.
[http://dx.doi.org/10.1111/bcp.12918] [PMID: 26914827]

[27]   Shrivastava AK, Singh HV, Raizada A, *et al.* Inflammatory markers in patients with rheumatoid arthritis. Allergol Immunopathol 2015; 43(1): 81-7.
[http://dx.doi.org/10.1016/j.aller.2013.11.003] [PMID: 24656623]

[28]   Sakhaei R, Shahvazi S, Mozaffari-Khosravi H, *et al.* The dietary approaches to stop hypertension (DASH)-Style diet and an alternative mediterranean diet are differently associated with serum inflammatory markers in female adults. food nutr bull 2018; 39(3): 361-76.
[http://dx.doi.org/10.1177/0379572118783950] [PMID: 29969908]

[29]   Soltani S, Chitsazi MJ, Salehi-Abargouei A. The effect of dietary approaches to stop hypertension (DASH) on serum inflammatory markers: A systematic review and meta-analysis of randomized trials. Clin Nutr 2018; 37(2): 542-50.
[http://dx.doi.org/10.1016/j.clnu.2017.02.018] [PMID: 28302405]

[30]   Melina V, Craig W, Levin S. Position of the academy of nutrition and dietetics: Vegetarian diets. J Acad Nutr Diet 2016; 116(12): 1970-80.
[http://dx.doi.org/10.1016/j.jand.2016.09.025] [PMID: 27886704]

[31]   Leitzmann C. Vegetarian diets: What are the advantages? Forum Nutr 2005; 57(57): 147-56.
[http://dx.doi.org/10.1159/000083787] [PMID: 15702597]

[32]   Li S, Micheletti R. Role of diet in rheumatic disease. Rheum Dis Clin North Am 2011; 37(1): 119-33.
[http://dx.doi.org/10.1016/j.rdc.2010.11.006] [PMID: 21220091]

[33]   Kjeldsen-Kragh J, Haugen M, Borchgrevink CF, *et al.* Controlled trial of fasting and one-year vegetarian diet in rheumatoid arthritis. Lancet 1991; 338(8772): 899-902.

[34]   Philippou E, Petersson SD, Rodomar C, Nikiphorou E. Rheumatoid arthritis and dietary interventions: systematic review of clinical trials. Nutr Rev 2021; 79(4): 410-28.
[http://dx.doi.org/10.1093/nutrit/nuaa033] [PMID: 32585000]

[35]   Huang RY, Huang CC, Hu FB, Chavarro JE. Vegetarian diets and weight reduction: A meta-analysis of randomized controlled trials. J Gen Intern Med 2016; 31(1): 109-16.
[http://dx.doi.org/10.1007/s11606-015-3390-7] [PMID: 26138004]

[36]   Athanassiou P, Athanassiou L, Kostoglou-Athanassiou I. Nutritional pearls: Diet and rheumatoid arthritis. Mediterr J Rheumatol 2020; 31(3): 319-24.
[http://dx.doi.org/10.31138/mjr.31.3.319] [PMID: 33163864]

[37] Alwarith J, Kahleova H, Rembert E, *et al.* Nutrition interventions in rheumatoid arthritis: The potential use of plant-based diets : A review. Front Nutr 2019; 6: 141.
[http://dx.doi.org/10.3389/fnut.2019.00141] [PMID: 31552259]

[38] Kim MS, Hwang SS, Park EJ, Bae JW. Strict vegetarian diet improves the risk factors associated with metabolic diseases by modulating gut microbiota and reducing intestinal inflammation. Environ Microbiol Rep 2013; 5(5).
[http://dx.doi.org/10.1111/1758-2229.12079] [PMID: 24115628]

[39] Philippou E, Nikiphorou E. Are we really what we eat? Nutrition and its role in the onset of rheumatoid arthritis. Autoimmun Rev 2018; 17(11): 1074-7.
[http://dx.doi.org/10.1016/j.autrev.2018.05.009] [PMID: 30213695]

[40] Ferraz-Amaro I, González-Juanatey C, López-Mejias R, Riancho-Zarrabeitia L, González-Gay MA. Metabolic syndrome in rheumatoid arthritis. Mediators Inflamm 2013; 2013: 1-11.
[http://dx.doi.org/10.1155/2013/710928] [PMID: 23431244]

[41] Lerner A, Freire de Carvalho J, Kotrova A, Shoenfeld Y. Gluten-free diet can ameliorate the symptoms of non-celiac autoimmune diseases. Nutr Rev 2022; 80(3): 525-43.
[http://dx.doi.org/10.1093/nutrit/nuab039] [PMID: 34338776]

[42] El-Chammas K, Danner E. Gluten-free diet in nonceliac disease. Nutr Clin Pract 2011; 26(3): 294-9.
[http://dx.doi.org/10.1177/0884533611405538] [PMID: 21586414]

[43] Elkan AC, Sjöberg B, Kolsrud B, Ringertz B, Hafström I, Frostegård J. Gluten-free vegan diet induces decreased LDL and oxidized LDL levels and raised atheroprotective natural antibodies against phosphorylcholine in patients with rheumatoid arthritis: A randomized study. Arthritis Res Ther 2008; 10(2): R34.
[http://dx.doi.org/10.1186/ar2388] [PMID: 18348715]

[44] Bruzzese V, Scolieri P, Pepe J. Efficacy of gluten-free diet in patients with rheumatoid arthritis. Reumatismo 2021; 72(4): 213-7.
[http://dx.doi.org/10.4081/reumatismo.2020.1296] [PMID: 33677948]

[45] Daien C, Czernichow S, Letarouilly JG, *et al.* Dietary recommendations of the french society for rheumatology for patients with chronic inflammatory rheumatic diseases. Joint Bone Spine 2022; 89(2): 105319.
[http://dx.doi.org/10.1016/j.jbspin.2021.105319] [PMID: 34902577]

[46] Malinowski B, Zalewska K, Węsierska A, *et al.* Intermittent fasting in cardiovascular disorders : An overview. Nutrients 2019; 11(3): 673.
[http://dx.doi.org/10.3390/nu11030673] [PMID: 30897855]

[47] Wang X, Yang Q, Liao Q, *et al.* Effects of intermittent fasting diets on plasma concentrations of inflammatory biomarkers: A systematic review and meta-analysis of randomized controlled trials. Nutrition 2020; 79-80: 110974.
[http://dx.doi.org/10.1016/j.nut.2020.110974] [PMID: 32947129]

[48] Longo VD, Mattson MP. Fasting: molecular mechanisms and clinical applications. Cell Metab 2014; 19(2): 181-92.
[http://dx.doi.org/10.1016/j.cmet.2013.12.008] [PMID: 24440038]

[49] Razavi R, Parvaresh A, Abbasi B, *et al.* The alternate-day fasting diet is a more effective approach than a calorie restriction diet on weight loss and hs-CRP levels. Int J Vitam Nutr Res 2021; 91(3-4): 242-50.
[http://dx.doi.org/10.1024/0300-9831/a000623] [PMID: 32003649]

[50] Dey M, Cutolo M, Nikiphorou E. Beverages in rheumatoid arthritis: What to prefer or to avoid. Nutrients 2020; 12(10): 3155.
[http://dx.doi.org/10.3390/nu12103155] [PMID: 33076469]

[51] Cuevas-Cervera M, Perez-Montilla JJ, Gonzalez-Muñoz A, Garcia-Rios MC, Navarro-Ledesma S. The

effectiveness of intermittent fasting, time restricted feeding, caloric restriction, a ketogenic diet and the mediterranean diet as part of the treatment plan to improve health and chronic musculoskeletal pain: A systematic review. Int J Environ Res Public Health 2022; 19(11): 6698.
[http://dx.doi.org/10.3390/ijerph19116698] [PMID: 35682282]

[52]   Häger J, Bang H, Hagen M, *et al.* The role of dietary fiber in rheumatoid arthritis patients: A feasibility study. Nutrients 2019; 11(10): 2392.
[http://dx.doi.org/10.3390/nu11102392] [PMID: 31591345]

[53]   Khanna S, Jaiswal KS, Gupta B. Managing rheumatoid arthritis with dietary interventions. Front Nutr 2017; 4: 52.
[http://dx.doi.org/10.3389/fnut.2017.00052] [PMID: 29167795]

[54]   Linos A, Kaklamani VG, Kaklamani E, *et al.* Dietary factors in relation to rheumatoid arthritis: A role for olive oil and cooked vegetables? Am J Clin Nutr 1999; 70(6): 1077-82.
[http://dx.doi.org/10.1093/ajcn/70.6.1077] [PMID: 10584053]

[55]   Hu Y, Sparks JA, Malspeis S, *et al.* Long-term dietary quality and risk of developing rheumatoid arthritis in women. Ann Rheum Dis 2017; 76(8): 1357-64.
[http://dx.doi.org/10.1136/annrheumdis-2016-210431] [PMID: 28137914]

[56]   Pitsavos C, Panagiotakos DB, Chrysohoou C, *et al.* The adoption of Mediterranean diet attenuates the development of acute coronary syndromes in people with the metabolic syndrome. Nutr J 2003; 2(1): 1.
[http://dx.doi.org/10.1186/1475-2891-2-1] [PMID: 12740043]

[57]   Ghavipour M, Sotoudeh G, Tavakoli E, Mowla K, Hasanzadeh J, Mazloom Z. Pomegranate extract alleviates disease activity and some blood biomarkers of inflammation and oxidative stress in Rheumatoid Arthritis patients. Eur J Clin Nutr 2017; 71(1): 92-6.
[http://dx.doi.org/10.1038/ejcn.2016.151] [PMID: 27577177]

[58]   Rondanelli M, Perdoni F, Peroni G, *et al.* Ideal food pyramid for patients with rheumatoid arthritis: A narrative review. Clin Nutr 2021; 40(3): 661-89.
[http://dx.doi.org/10.1016/j.clnu.2020.08.020] [PMID: 32928578]

[59]   Tedeschi S, Bathon J, Giles J, Lin T-C, Yoshida K, Solomon D. The relationship between fish consumption and disease activity in rheumatoid arthritis. Arthritis Care Res 2017; 70.

[60]   Pedersen M, Stripp C, Klarlund M, Olsen SF, Tjønneland AM, Frisch M. Diet and risk of rheumatoid arthritis in a prospective cohort. J Rheumatol 2005; 32(7): 1249-52.
[PMID: 15996059]

[61]   Hagfors L, Nilsson I, Sköldstam L, Johansson G. Fat intake and composition of fatty acids in serum phospholipids in a randomized, controlled, Mediterranean dietary intervention study on patients with rheumatoid arthritis. Nutr Metab 2005; 2(1): 26.
[http://dx.doi.org/10.1186/1743-7075-2-26] [PMID: 16216119]

[62]   Salliot C, Nguyen Y, Boutron-Ruault MC, Seror R. Environment and Lifestyle: Their Influence on the Risk of RA. J Clin Med 2020; 9(10): 3109.
[http://dx.doi.org/10.3390/jcm9103109] [PMID: 32993091]

[63]   Schwingshackl L, Christoph M, Hoffmann G. Effects of olive oil on markers of inflammation and endothelial function : A systematic review and meta-analysis. Nutrients 2015; 7(9): 7651-75.
[http://dx.doi.org/10.3390/nu7095356] [PMID: 26378571]

[64]   Pattison DJ, Symmons DPM, Lunt M, *et al.* Dietary risk factors for the development of inflammatory polyarthritis: Evidence for a role of high level of red meat consumption. Arthritis Rheum 2004; 50(12): 3804-12.
[http://dx.doi.org/10.1002/art.20731] [PMID: 15593211]

[65]   Sundström B, Ljung L, Di Giuseppe D. Consumption of meat and dairy products is not associated with the risk for rheumatoid arthritis among women: A population-based cohort study. Nutrients 2019;

11(11): 2825.
[http://dx.doi.org/10.3390/nu11112825] [PMID: 31752273]

[66]   Benito-Garcia E, Feskanich D, Hu FB, Mandl LA, Karlson EW. Protein, iron, and meat consumption and risk for rheumatoid arthritis: A prospective cohort study. Arthritis Res Ther 2007; 9(1): R16.
[http://dx.doi.org/10.1186/ar2123] [PMID: 17288585]

[67]   He J, Wang Y, Feng M, *et al.* Dietary intake and risk of rheumatoid arthritis—a cross section multicenter study. Clin Rheumatol 2016; 35(12): 2901-8.
[http://dx.doi.org/10.1007/s10067-016-3383-x] [PMID: 27553386]

CHAPTER 7

Self-perceived Quality of Life in South Asian and British White Rheumatoid Arthritis Patients in the East Midlands, UK

A.M. Ghelani[1], A. Moorthy[2], L. Goh[2], A. Samanta[2], Puneetpal Singh[3] and Sarabjit Mastana[1,*]

[1] Human Genetics Lab., School of Sport, Exercise and Health Sciences, Loughborough University, Loughborough, LE11 3TU, United Kingdom

[2] Rheumatology, University Hospitals of Leicester NHS Trust, Leicester, United Kingdom

[3] Department of Human Genetics, Punjabi University, Patiala, Punjab, India

Abstract: It has been suggested that South Asian patients with RA report increased levels of pain and demonstrated increased disease severity as compared to the British *white* population. This study assesses the self-perceived quality of life in South Asian RA patients compared to White British RA patients. 131 South Asian (SA) and 134 British White (BW) RA patients from the East Midlands participated in the study as a part of ongoing studies on RA pathogenesis by completing the qualitative lifestyle questionnaire. The SA patients developed RA significantly earlier than BW patients (χ^2 = 21.01, P = 0.001, df = 5). Compared to the BW, a majority of SA perceived the disease to be severe (χ^2 = 8.57, P < 0.05, df = 3). They also reported higher pain (χ^2 = 26.12, P < 0.05, df = 3), reduced mobility (χ^2 = 17.57, P < 0.004, df = 5) and reduced physical activity performed (χ^2 = 17.94, P < 0.0005, df = 3). Reduced mobility and a decrease in physical activity may be associated with a higher perception of RA-related pain among South Asians. This may have important public health implications in terms of disease progression and treatment modalities.

Keywords: QoL, South Asian, British White, Rheumatoid Arthritis.

INTRODUCTION

Rheumatoid Arthritis (RA) is a chronic, multi-system disease with a considerable impact on the lives of individuals and their families. RA affects approximately 1% of the adult population. The East Midlands of the UK is an area with a substantial South Asian population. To optimise care, it is important to gather specific infor-

* **Corresponding author Sarabjit Mastana:** Human Genetics Lab., School of Sport, Exercise and Health Sciences, Loughborough University, Loughborough, LE11 3TU, United Kingdom; Tel: +44-7891-068708; E-mail: s.s.mastana@lboro.ac.uk

mation about this group of patients. The government initiative to provide equality in healthcare because of the Race Relations Amendment Act 2000 [1] and the King's Fund recommendation [2] suggests that ethnically specific data needs to be collected across the NHS to optimise healthcare. This would include obtaining and responding effectively to the patients 'raw feelings' (patients' perception of the disease treatment following the confirmatory diagnosis of RA). Quality of life (QoL) measures are equally important to measure in chronic disease management and this may reflect on patient satisfaction. In other words, if patients perceive that their quality of life is at a reasonable level then it may follow that they have greater satisfaction and (possibly confidence) in their current treatment. The beneficial effects on their health may reflect this, in the longer term.

Both environmental and genetic factors have been documented to play a significant role in the pathogenesis of RA. However, measures of disease activity and disease damage are insufficient to fully assess the impact of RA on an individual. This aspect is also important to clinicians in assessing the benefits of prescribed medications. There are only a few studies on patients from South Asia (India, Sri Lanka and Pakistan) with RA on this aspect and no comparative studies have been published [3]. These studies have used health-related quality of life (HRQoL) questionnaires reflecting patients' subjective evaluation of the effects of disease on their physical, psychological and social functioning. Studies on RA QOL have clearly documented that RA has a profound effect on the functioning and well-being of patients [3]. While HRQOL and other QoL instruments are useful tools, all have limitations. These questionnaires tend to be detailed, take a long time to complete, and have limited availability of validated translated versions. The translated questionnaires often do not convey the correct interpretation and have poorly translated terminologies that ethnic minorities may have difficulties comprehending, resulting in problems in the completion of the questionnaires. The current validated questionnaires often fail to assess 'raw feelings' [4], in relation to out-patient complaints, which may prove to be a more sensitive measure for what needs to be altered (if at all) within clinical practice. In this study, we have assessed patients' perception of quality of life (QoL) amongst hospital-referred South Asian (SA) and British White (BW) RA patients from the East Midlands by means of a questionnaire. We hypothesized that both groups would have similar perceptions of QoL as all participants are from the same geographical area, share similar environmental features, and have similar accessibility to health services. In this questionnaire, we specifically focused on the perception of pain and severity, disability, and medications.

METHODS

Rheumatoid factor-positive RA patients between the age of 20 and 75 years participated in the QoL assessment; all fulfilled the ACR 1987 criteria for RA [5]. A self-administered questionnaire written in the English language was used in the study. Complete access to appropriate interpretation/translation facility was available to all participants. The questionnaire was piloted to assess the suitability and understanding of questions among participants, some questions were reworded to avoid any confusion. The questionnaire consisted of questions related to personal information (age, gender, marital status, ethnicity, family status, occupation, diet, cigarette and alcohol consumption, exercise, duration of disease, self-perceived severity of disease and pain, and medications). Patients were requested to indicate mild, moderate or severe state of daily pain and RA status, mobility and amount of daily exercise performed in hours. The effect of other 'raw feelings' on the scoring was monitored by providing a facility in the questionnaire to comment on any other aspects of the disease. The progression of RA in the two ethnic groups was calculated by deducting the age of the patient at the time of answering the questionnaire from the confirmed onset of the disease at the RA clinic.

About 10% of participants were asked to complete the questionnaire on more than one occasion to ascertain whether they provided the same responses and a degree of internal validity in responses.

The study received Loughborough University Ethics Committee and NHS approval and all subjects gave written informed consent. SPSS (Version 15.0.1) was used for statistical analysis.

RESULTS

131 South Asian (M = 28, F = 103) and 134 British White (M = 36, F = 98) participants successfully completed the questionnaires. Most South Asian participants were migrants mainly from India and composed of Gujarati and Punjabi groups. Some Gujarati participants migrated to the UK from East Africa (Kenya, Uganda and Tanzania). Britsh White participants were natives from the East Midlands of the UK.

Age and Gender Distribution

The mean age of SA patients was 52.5 years (Standard deviation (S.D.) of 10.3 years, n = 131) and BW was 58.9 years (S.D. 10.3 years, n = 134). The difference was statistically significant (t = 5.10, P<0.0001). Age distribution (Fig. **1**) showed that there were more SA-RA patients (41%) in the age range of 31 to 50 years as compared to BW (20%), leading to statistically significant differences ($\chi^2 = 21.01$, df = 5, P = 0.001). South Asian RA age distribution was skewed towards a younger population (Fig. **1**). There was differential gender distribution in the two groups (M:F 1:3.7 in SA and 1:2.7 in BW).

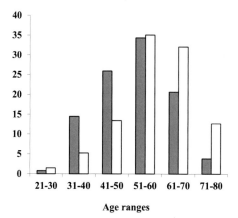

Fig. (1). Age distribution in South Asian (filled bars) and British White (unfilled bars) RA patients. Y-axis shows percentage count of each age group.

Age of Onset and Duration of Disease

There were no significant differences between the two ethnic groups in terms of the age of onset which occurred before the age of 50 years. In both groups, the duration of disease ranged from 2 years to 50 years. Approximately 1/3 of South Asians (34%) were in the 6 - 10 years duration of disease range (Fig. **2**).

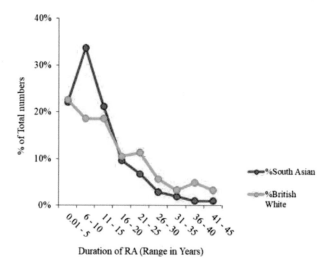

Fig. (2). Duration of RA in South Asian and British White patients.

Severity and Pain Perception

There was a significant difference in the perception of disease severity among SA and BW RA patients (χ^2 = 8.57, P < 0.05, df = 3). More South Asian RA patients considered their RA status to be of moderate to severe severity compared to BW patients. A similar pattern was observed in pain perception (Fig. **3**). More SA patients reported severe pain compared to BW patients (χ^2 = 26.12, P < 0.05, df = 3). These results provide some support to anecdotal clinical observations that South Asian patients report higher levels of severity and pain [6, 7].

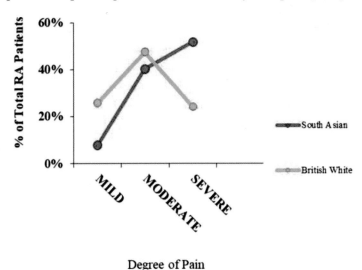

Fig. (3). Degree of Pain perception in South Asian and British White RA patients.

As expected, there was a significant association between the pain and the severity of RA in both groups (χ^2 = 118.43, P < 0.001, df = 4 in South Asians and χ^2 = 75.47, P < 0.001, df = 4 in British Whites) indicating that higher severity led to higher pain perception. Contrary to the common belief that older RA patients report higher pain perception, there was no association between age and pain perception (P > 0.05) in any group in this study [8].

Mobility and Exercise

South Asian patients reported reduced mobility (χ^2 = 17.57, P < 0.004, df = 5) and restricted their exercise activities to less than one hour per day. BW patients were fairly mobile. There was a significant difference in the amount of physical activity performed between the two groups (χ^2 = 17.94, P < 0.0005, df = 3).

Medications

Aspirin, steroids, DMARDs, or a combination of these drugs were the primary medications for a majority of RA patients. There was a good match between the length of medication and the duration of disease in both groups. BW patients were more likely to be on aspirin, NSAIDs, and steroid medications, while more South Asians were prescribed methotrexate and other DMARDS. It was not possible to separate sufficiently all the treatment groups due to undergoing multiple drug therapy.

Other Lifestyle Aspects

There were more office and manual workers in BW patients, whilst the majority of South Asians, and females were housewives. There were more vegetarians among SA patients compared to BW patients who were mostly non-vegetarian. Smoking was reported by a small number of participants and did not lead to any significant difference between groups (7% SA and 14% BW). South Asian RA male patients reported low/occasional consumption of alcohol while BW patients reported regular consumption.

DISCUSSION

This is the first report on self-perceptions of the quality of life in South Asian RA patients of the East Midlands, UK. The analyses document that South Asian patients experience more pain and reduced quality of life than British White patients. The reasons for this may have important implications if we are to improve treatment outcomes in this group. The main findings of the data analyses suggest that South Asian patients perceive their rheumatoid arthritis to be of moderate to severe severity, that they have a higher level of pain, and have reduced mobility and physical activity levels.

A number of biological and cultural factors (*e.g.,* culture, education, support, diet, and medications) may lead to differential perceptions of pain and severity among different populations. Some studies on South Asians have reported that musculoskeletal pain is more generalised [9]. There is also well-documented evidence that the low level of vitamin D contributes to the widespread pain among South Asians [10 - 15]. As vitamin D levels were not measured directly in this study, it is difficult to directly link pain, and disease severity with possible lower vitamin D levels among South Asian RA patients.

A greater number of South Asians compared to British Whites reported reduced mobility and were either wheelchair bound, restricted to the home, or required support during walking, indicating a greater deterioration of quality of life in the

South Asian group. It is highly unlikely that cultural differences contributed to the reduced mobility as reported in a study [16], since, the severity of RA and pain were perceived to be significantly associated with each other in the present study.

In this study, more South Asian RA patients were reported to be on DMARD than BW patients. This is an interesting observation as in some previous studies it has been reported that South Asian patients are less tolerant of DMARDs and stopped the use of these therapies earlier than North Europeans [17]. Helliwell and colleagues [17] reported rashes, lack of efficacy, and side effects to be the primary reasons for discontinuation of DMARD therapies among South Asians. As the emerging concept of management of RA is to treat the disease very early and aggressively, it may be that it was considered reasonable to introduce DMARDS therapy earlier in South Asia, as is partly reflected in our study.

The detailed self-reporting questionnaire used in the study was designed following advice from local doctors and the community and was found to be the most suitable for including the raw feelings of the patients. It has a face value but as a novel questionnaire, it may be criticised for its lack of evaluation. Further work is required to evaluate the questionnaire. However, some participants (~10%) also completed this questionnaire on more than one occasion and provided the same responses demonstrating reproducibility in responses. Overall our results and observations match well with previous studies which also document that South Asian patients report higher pain and disability than patients of North European origin [17, 18].

Further comprehensive studies are required to confirm if the age distribution differences observed in this study were due to chance or population demography or early onset of disease among South Asians. Similar early progression to disease status has been reported for other complex diseases such as diabetes, heart disease and hypertension amongst South Asians in the UK and other Western countries. As with any volunteer-based disease analysis study, there was a lack of participation of all age groups (especially the late age group) among South Asians due to disability, lack of interest, and cultural and religious reasons which may have contributed to differences in age distribution among two groups.

There were significantly higher numbers of South Asian patients under the age of 50 while the age of onset was similar in both groups. These differences could be due to genetic or environmental factors which may predispose the South Asian group to develop the disease earlier and also increase the severity and usage of DMARDS earlier than other populations.

Overall this study documents that there are distinct differences in perceptions of pain, disability, and severity related to RA among South Asians and British White patients which may require different treatment regimens and management strategies. Some of these differences could be biological, nutritional and other factors. It's important for individuals with RA to work closely with their healthcare providers to develop an individualized treatment plan that addresses their specific needs and goals. It's also important to remember that every person is different and may have different perceptions, preferences, and needs, so it's important to personalize the RA treatments using a combination of medications, physical therapy, occupational therapy, pain management, exercise, counseling and diet and nutrition to improve the quality of life.

CONCLUSION

The results of the present study document that South Asian RAs report higher levels of severity and pain which may have implications for clinical treatments and disease management by medical practitioners. Reduced mobility may be associated with higher perception of pain by this group. This study also shows that contrary to common belief that older RA patients complain of more pain, this study did not find any association between age, duration of disease, and pain perception. Personalised treatment and management strategies are required to support the quality of life for RA patients in different populations which should also take into consideration the nutritional, cultural and perceptual needs of an individual patient.

REFERENCES

[1]   Race relations (Amendment) Act. Implementing good practice. 2000. Available from: http://www.nta.nhs.uk/publications/documents/nta_race_relations_section7.1.pdf

[2]   Stanley E. Working to Sustain Progress: Black and minority ethnic non-executive directors in London. 1st., Kings fund publications 2006.

[3]   Bedi GS, Gupta N, Handa R, Pal H, Pandey RM. Quality of life in Indian patients with rheumatoid arthritis. Qual Life Res 2005; 14(8): 1953-8.
[http://dx.doi.org/10.1007/s11136-005-4540-x] [PMID: 16155783]

[4]   Walker A. Watchdog urges NHS to learn from "raw feelings of patients" in report on 16,000 complaints. 2007. Available from: https://www.ivyroses.com/Health/1622#:~:text=1%20February%202007-,Watchdog%20urges%20NHS%20to%20learn%20from%20%22raw%20feelings%20of%20patients,in%20report%20on%2016%2C000%20complaints&text=The%20Healthcare%20Commission%20is%20urging,quickly%2C%20efficiently%20and%20locally%E2%80%9D

[5]   Arnett FC, Edworthy SM, Bloch DA, *et al*. The american rheumatism association 1987 revised criteria for the classification of rheumatoid arthritis. Arthritis Rheum 1988; 31(3): 315-24.
[http://dx.doi.org/10.1002/art.1780310302] [PMID: 3358796]

[6]   Palmer B, Macfarlane G, Afzal C, Esmail A, Silman A, Lunt M. Acculturation and the prevalence of pain amongst South Asian minority ethnic groups in the UK. Rheumatology 2007; 46(6): 1009-14.
[http://dx.doi.org/10.1093/rheumatology/kem037] [PMID: 17401133]

[7]   Afzal CW, Finn JD, Lunt M, *et al*. Acculturation is associated with a reduction in chronic widespread pain in persons of South Asian origin in the United Kingdom. Br J Rheumatol 2002; 41: 2-2.

[8] Hameed K, Gibson T. A comparison of the prevalence of rheumatoid arthritis and other rheumatic diseases amongst Pakistanis living in England and Pakistan. Rheumatology 1997; 36(7): 781-5.
[http://dx.doi.org/10.1093/rheumatology/36.7.781] [PMID: 9255114]

[9] Young M, Baar K. Women and Pain: Why It Hurts and What You Can Do. Boston, USA: Hyperion Books 2002; pp. 23-124.

[10] Allison TR, Symmons DPM, Brammah T, *et al.* Musculoskeletal pain is more generalised among people from ethnic minorities than among white people in Greater Manchester. Ann Rheum Dis 2002; 61(2): 151-6.
[http://dx.doi.org/10.1136/ard.61.2.151] [PMID: 11796402]

[11] Macfarlane GJ, Palmer B, Roy D, Afzal C, Silman AJ, O'Neill T. An excess of widespread pain among South Asians: are low levels of vitamin D implicated? Ann Rheum Dis 2005; 64(8): 1217-9.
[http://dx.doi.org/10.1136/ard.2004.032656] [PMID: 16014682]

[12] Hamson C, Goh L, Sheldon P, Samanta A. Comparative study of bone mineral density, calcium, and vitamin D status in the Gujarati and white populations of Leicester. Postgrad Med J 2003; 79(931): 279-83.
[http://dx.doi.org/10.1136/pmj.79.931.279] [PMID: 12782775]

[13] Serhan E, Holland MR. Relationship of hypovitaminosis D and secondary hyperparathyroidism with bone mineral density among UK resident Indo-Asians. Ann Rheum Dis 2002; 61(5): 456-8.
[http://dx.doi.org/10.1136/ard.61.5.456] [PMID: 11959772]

[14] Serhan E, Holland MR. Calcium and vitamin D supplementation failed to improve bone mineral density in Indo-Asians suffering from hypovitaminosis D and secondary hyperparathyroidism. Rheumatol Int 2005; 25(4): 276-9.
[http://dx.doi.org/10.1007/s00296-003-0430-0] [PMID: 14727056]

[15] Goh L, Samanta A, Hamson C, Badhesha J, Sheldon P. Bone mineral density: Calcium and vitamin D status in Gujarati and Punjabi South Asians in Leicester. Practical evidence 2006; 2: 4-12.

[16] Netto G, McCloughan L, Bhatnagar A. Effective heart disease prevention: Lessons from a qualitative study of user perspectives in Bangladeshi, Indian and Pakistani communities. Public Health 2007; 121(3): 177-86.
[http://dx.doi.org/10.1016/j.puhe.2006.11.001] [PMID: 17224165]

[17] Helliwell PS, Ibrahim G. Ethnic differences in responses to disease modifying drugs. Br J Rheumatol 2003; 42(10): 1197-201.
[http://dx.doi.org/10.1093/rheumatology/keg354] [PMID: 12810940]

[18] Griffiths B, Situnayake RD, Clark B, Tennant A, Salmon M, Emery P. Racial origin and its effect on disease expression and HLA-DRB1 types in patients with rheumatoid arthritis: A matched cross-sectional study. Rheumatology 2000; 39(8): 857-64.
[http://dx.doi.org/10.1093/rheumatology/39.8.857] [PMID: 10952739]

SUBJECT INDEX

A

ACE inhibitors 85
Acid, uric 3
Acidic 47, 52
    enzymes 47
    phosphoprotein 52
Actin cytoskeleton 47
Activation 8, 31, 33, 34, 35, 36, 54, 56, 85
    cytokine 36
    monocyte 31, 35
    renin-angiotensin-aldosterone system 85
    synovial fibroblast 35
Activity, osteoclastic 87
Adaptive immune systems 31, 55
Ageing 75, 76, 77, 78, 80, 81, 82, 83, 85, 86
    population 82
    skeleton 82
Agent, regulatory 57
Aging 5, 75, 82, 86
    -induced bone porosity 82
AI-assisted methods 18
Air pollution 96
Alanine amino-transferase 7
Alcohol 5, 6, 116
    consumption 6, 116
    intake 6
    metabolism 5
Algorithm-based machine learning 18
Alkaline phosphatase 47
Allergic rhinitis 57
AMP-activated protein kinase 63
Angiogenesis 33, 37
Angiotensin 8, 85
Anteroposterior radiograph 21
Anti-citrullinated peptide antibodies (ACPA) 40
Anti-cyclic citrullinated peptide 61
Anti-inflammatory 9, 99
    cytokine profile 9
    process 99
Anti-rheumatic 39, 62

dugs 62
effective 39
Antigen-presenting cells (APCs) 56
Antioxidants 101, 102
Antiviral treatment 3
APC activity 58
Arthritis 32, 33, 37, 51, 61, 62, 98
Atheroprotective 104
Autoimmune 1, 2, 4, 5, 6, 35, 40, 52, 53, 54, 56, 59, 96
    disorders 35, 52, 59
    illnesses 35, 53, 54, 56
    inflammatory process 96
    liver diseases (ALD) 1, 2, 4, 5, 6
    thyroiditis 40
Autoimmune diseases 10, 31, 40, 62, 105
    chronic 31

B

Blood 2, 40, 49, 87
    glucose levels, lowering 87
    virus-infected 2
Bone 3, 7, 9, 39, 41, 46, 47, 48, 49, 51, 52, 56, 59, 60, 75, 76, 77, 78, 81, 83, 84, 85, 86, 87, 88, 96
    alkaline phosphatase 3
    blood flow 81
    deformities 46, 49, 59
    degradation 39, 41, 96
    diseases 46, 75, 88
    dried 78
    erosion 56
    health, regulating 48, 49
    homeostasis 46, 48
    hydration 75, 76, 77, 78, 86, 87
    loading, prolonged 78
    mammalian 76
    marrow cells 56
    mechanical properties of 83, 85, 87
    metabolism 7, 46, 48
    microdamage 78